Eat It or Drink It

How to boost your health and manage your weight using fruits, vegetables and other superfoods *(Recipes included)*

NATHALIE D. TALOM

Disclaimer:

The information in this book is designed to maintain good health and does not claim to diagnose or cure any disease. If you are pregnant, breastfeeding, or you are on any medication, please check with your health care provider before making any changes to your diet.

Eat It or Drink It: *How to boost your health using fruits, vegetables and other superfoods*

ISBN-13: 978-0692928349
ISBN-10: 0692928340

Library of Congress Control Number: 2017913673
Nathalie Talom, Midland, TX

Cover Design by Jedidiah Talom

Cover photo by Jedidiah Talom

Published in the United States of America

01   02   03   04   05   06   07   08   09   10

Table of Contents

INTRODUCTION---
----1

CHAPTER ONE
    HOW DID WE GET HERE? -------------------------------------
------3

CHAPTER TWO
    PROCESSED VS. WHOLE FOODS----------------------------
-----15

CHAPTER THREE
    RECLAIMING YOUR HEALTH----------------------------------
-----27

CHAPTER FOUR
    NATURE'S "MIRACLE PILLS" ----------------------------------
------33

CHAPTER FIVE
    IF YOU CAN'T EAT THEM, DRINK THEM---------------------
-----41

CHAPTER SIX
    HEALTH BENEFITS OF SUPERFOOD SMOOTHIES-------------
----47

CHAPTER SEVEN

LEAFY GREENS & OTHER VEGETABLES----------------------
-----55

CHAPTER EIGHT
WHAT FRUITS TO USE-------------------------------------
-----75

CHAPTER NINE
SUPERFOOD SMOOTHIE 101------------------------------
-----85

CHAPTER TEN
PROTEIN IN YOUR SMOOTHIE-----------------------------
-----91

CHAPTER ELEVEN
SUPER-CHARGE YOUR SMOOTHIE WITH SUPERFOODS-----
---103

CHAPTER TWELVE
TIPS FOR A GREAT SMOOTHIE EXPERIENCE------------------
----127

CHAPTER THIRTEEN
BLENDING VS. JUICING----------------------------------
----135

CHAPTER FOURTEEN
JUICING 101---
----141

CHAPTER FIFTEEN
SUPERFOODS AND THEIR BENEFITS-------------------------
---153

CHAPTER SIXTEEN

CONCLUSION---

---161

RECIPES

NATHALIE'S SMOOTHIE FAVORITES---------------------------

---163

NATHALIE'S JUICING FAVORITES-----------------------------

---173

10-DAY RESET PLAN--

----179

Introduction

❖❖❖❖❖❖

I f you came home one day and noticed that your kitchen floor was flooded, would you simply clean up the mess, without identifying the cause? I don't think so! You would be more likely to put a bucket or towel at the source of the leak, and then attempt to determine the cause. In that way, you would not have to rely on a temporary fix to avoid such a problem in the future.

If you are comfortable with a temporary solution, however, and ignore the need to address the cause, you will be faced with the inconvenience of emptying a bucket and wringing out towels, on a regular basis. You could also run the risk of not only a flooded kitchen, but the problem spreading throughout the house, causing damage to furniture and carpets, etc.

When it comes to our health, the same thing is true. Our society today is facing a major health crisis of chronic condition, such as obesity, high blood pressure, heart disease, Type 2 diabetes, auto-immune diseases, and cancer—to name just a few. Unfortunately, medications have not proven to be effective in curing most of these conditions. They have simply minimized the symptoms. Sadly enough, instead of looking at the root causes, of such chronic health problems, society has chosen to look to doctors, and prescribed drugs that offer an easy approach to managing the symptoms. This is simply putting a bucket under a leak. It can cause more damage than the initial problem.

This book is intended to outline the progression of chronic disease in our society, as well as identify some of the root causes. It also suggests ways to address issues at the root—nutritionally poor diets. It is my hope that this information inspires, and equips, you, to become an active participant in your own health goals, by making it fun and easy to eat whole foods that nourish your body.

Remember, your health is a key asset to fulfilling your dreams. Nevertheless, it is your responsibility to fiercely fight for it!

Chapter One
How Did We Get Here?

❖❖❖❖❖❖

O ver the past few decades, the medical profession has made incredible strides in preventing and combatting medical problems. As a population, however, we are becoming sicker. At the beginning of the 20th century, infectious diseases were what killed people. Nowadays, chronic diseases are the primary cause of death and disability in the Unites States. This has been the case since the late 1900s, as revealed on the following graphs.

1900

Cause	(bar chart, Percentage 0–40)
Pneumonia	
Tuberculosis	
Diarrhea and Enteritis	
Heart Disease	
Stroke	
Liver Disease	
Injuries	
Cancer	
Senility	
Diphtheria	

Percentage

1997

Cause	(bar chart, Percentage 0–40)
Heart Disease	
Cancer	
Stroke	
Chronic Lung Disease	
Unintentional Injury	
Pneumonia and Influenza	
Diabetes	
HIV Infection	
Suicide	
Chronic Liver Disease	

Percentage

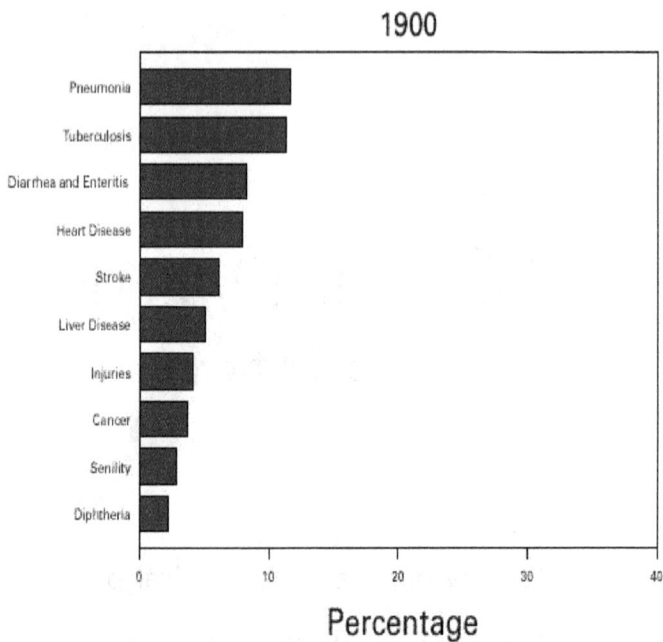

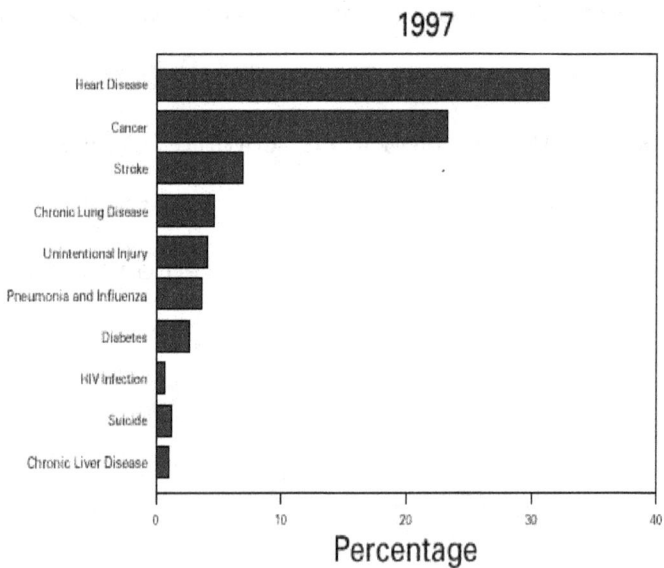

Figure 1: Leading causes of death as a percentage of all death - United States, 1990 and 1997

4

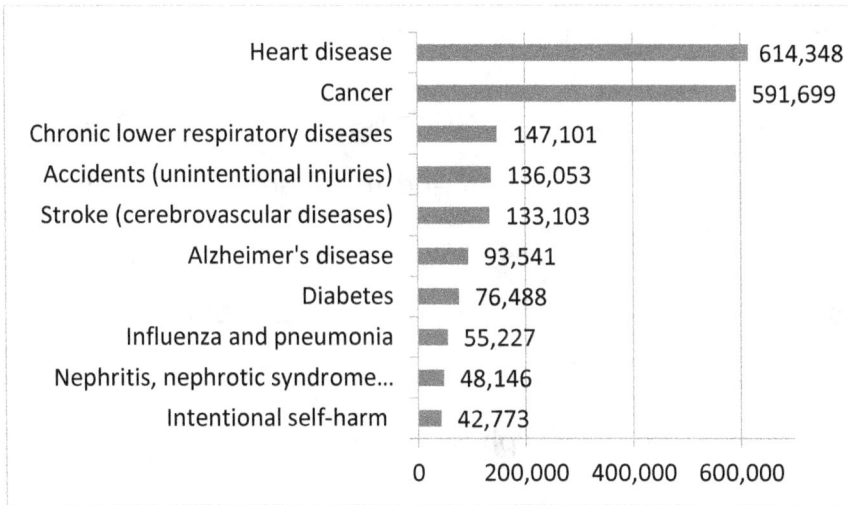

Cause	Deaths
Heart disease	614,348
Cancer	591,699
Chronic lower respiratory diseases	147,101
Accidents (unintentional injuries)	136,053
Stroke (cerebrovascular diseases)	133,103
Alzheimer's disease	93,541
Diabetes	76,488
Influenza and pneumonia	55,227
Nephritis, nephrotic syndrome...	48,146
Intentional self-harm	42,773

0   200,000   400,000   600,000

Figure 2: Leading cause of death in the United States in 2014

Data Source: http://www.cdc.gov/nchs/fastats/leading-causes-of-death.htm

The high rate of chronic diseases today, along with the decrease in epidemic, infectious diseases, raise the question; "How did we move from an epidemic of infectious diseases to an epidemic of chronic disease in the last century?"

First let's look at the difference between the two types of disease.

Infectious disease is a disease caused by a bug such as bacteria, viruses, parasites, or fungi. The onset is rapid and the duration is often short. Chronic disease, on the other hand, is not normally caused in such a manner, except in some cases such as of HIV.

The onset is slow and the affected person can suffer with the disease for a long period of time, ranging from months to years.

According to the Centers for Disease Control and Prevention (CDC), a small set of common and modifiable, risk factors are responsible for most of the main, chronic conditions, such as obesity, heart disease, cancer, stroke, high blood pressure, chronic respiratory disease, and Type 2 diabetes. Some of these risk factors are poor diet, physical inactivity, tobacco use, and excess alcohol consumption.

http://www.cdc.gov/chronicdisease/overview/

Many efforts, by both the government and individuals, have been made to decrease the rate of these risk factors; however, unfortunately, our poor diet remains a serious concern. It leads us to the question, "What has changed in our diet that could have contributed to this health disaster?"

It has been determined that the primary change is that we went from a whole food diet to a highly processed and fast food diet. In days past, our ancestors ate what they grew, or purchased, from farms. In the mid-nineteen hundred's, however, changes in societal behavior led to the proliferation of processed and fast foods. This has now become the staple of the American diet.

As early as 1910, processed foods were beginning to appear—Nathan's hot dogs, Aunt Jemima syrup, Hellmann's mayonnaise, Oreo cookies, Crisco, and Marshmallow Fluff, to name just a few. These were followed by many more in the next few decades. The first fast food chain, White Castle, opened in 1921, followed, in 1930, by Kentucky Fried Chicken, and McDonalds in 1940. Homemade meals from fresh produce, however, were still the staple of our diet, until after World War II. This was when American eating habits truly began to change. Rationale for these changes includes:

- Labor shortage during World War II

During World War II (1939-1945), men went off to war in large numbers, and this caused a labor shortage, forcing women to join the workforce like never before. As this occurred, women's busy schedules made it increasingly convenient to have a meal that was readily available than to cook one from scratch. Furthermore, the feminist movement of the 1960s encouraged even more women to work outside of the home. Thus, further increased the demand for quick and easy meals. This habit was also driven by escalating TV ads promoting the convenience of household microwave ovens, introduced in 1967. Frozen dinners, canned foods, and fast foods became the ultimate solution to a busy lifestyle and were well received by the population. Following the War, processed food and fast food restaurants were available everywhere, and people started to eat out on a regular basis.

- ## The modernization of farming

During World War II, there was also a revolution in science that expedited the production of materials and supplies needed to support the war. Many of these new technologies were also used to develop modern machinery utilized in agricultural efforts. Not only did these new technologies improve the processing and transportation of food for the soldiers, it contributed to the introduction of more processed food for the general public. This switch from traditional agricultural practices to more modern methods of production further included a greater use of chemicals, such as pesticides, herbicides, and synthetic fertilizers. While they were intended to support an enhanced production of food unfortunately, in many cases, these new trends had a negative effect on some farming practices. A heightened demand for meat often resulted in factory-type farming that poorly impacted living conditions for animals, and an increased use of antibiotics and hormones, to boost production.

- Government politics

In response to increasing demands for food products, the government initiated a policy of subsidizing expanded production of corn, wheat, soybeans, and meat. This further contributed to the proliferation of fast and processed foods, by cutting production costs. Lowered production costs, and increased competition within the fast food industry, led to a practice of increased serving sizes, as seen in the data below. More calories per meal was the outcome. When compared to other countries, the serving size of American fast foods is outrageous. Studies have proven that excess calories lead to obesity and many of the chronic illnesses we are dealing with today.

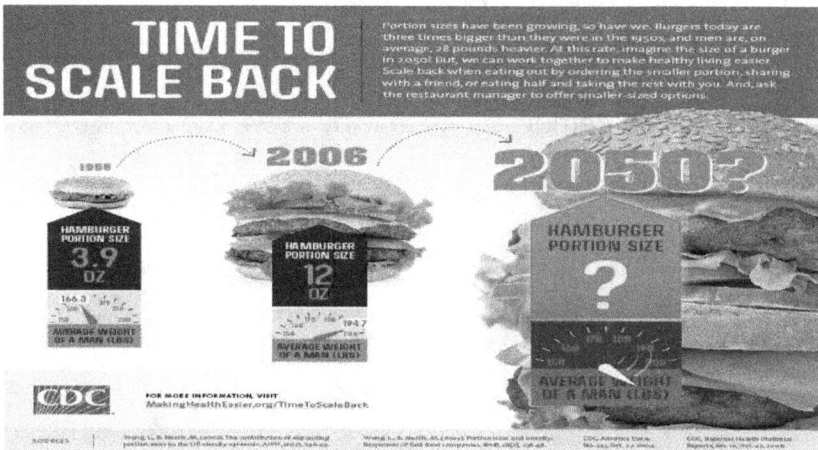

Figure 3: Evolution of fast food portion size over the years

Source: CDC

9

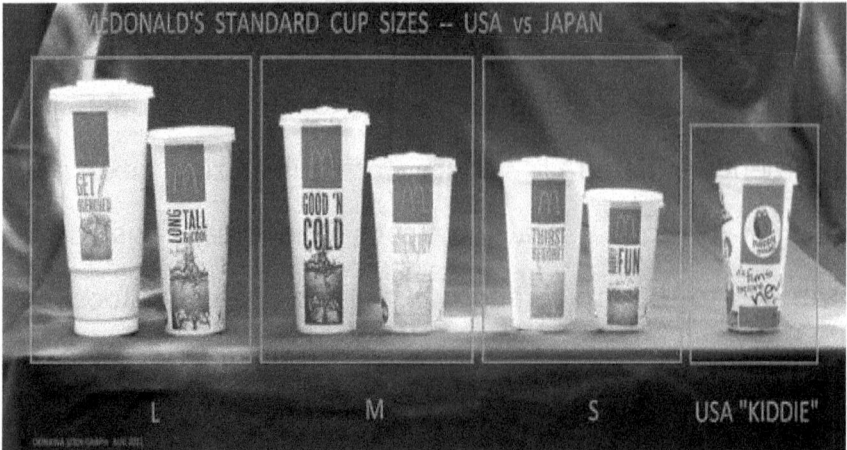

Figure 4: Comparison of McDonald's standard cups sizes USA vs Japan

Source: https://www.flickr.com/photos/okinawa-soba/6004485662/in/album-72157627220835741/

These changes were subtle and took place without public attention. People were pleased by faster, cheaper, and more food at the same price. Unfortunately, they had no idea that their health was being negatively affected, until the 1970s, when waist lines started to increase. Obesity became a public health concern. The graph below demonstrates that by 1994, the rate of obesity had risen significantly, compared to the mid-nineteen hundreds. In fact, it has been increasing ever since—setting the stage for an epidemic of chronic disease, as we see today.

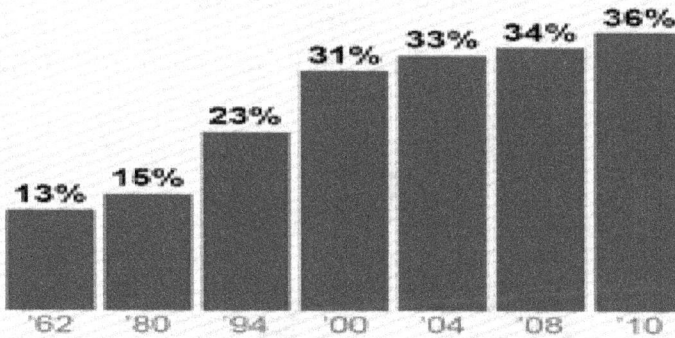

Obesity over time
Percentage of obese adults, ages 20 to 74:

Source: Centers for Disease Control and Prevention
By Frank Pompa, USA TODAY

Figure 5: Evolution of obesity rate in the USA from 1962-2010

Source: USA Today website

Even childhood obesity, once rare, has flourished. In 2011-2014, the prevalence of obesity had reached 8.9% among 2 to 5-year old's, 17.5% among 6 to 11-year old's, and 20.5% among 12 to 19-year old's.

https://www.cdc.gov/obesity/data/childhood.html

It has also been confirmed, by many studies, that plaque buildup in the arteries can actually have its beginnings in childhood. This predisposes children to be affected, of such conditions as heart disease, into adulthood. As we mentioned earlier, heart disease is the number one killer disease, in the United States today. Experts predict that, if nothing is done about our diets soon, our children might be the first generation of Americans to have a shorter life expectancy than their parents. Parents, therefore, must keep in mind that, what is on a child's plate today, can radically impact his/her health tomorrow.

- **The effect of GMOs on our diet**

We can't talk about the changes that have affected the way we eat, however, without mentioning the introduction of genetically, modified organisms (GMOs) in the farming process today. A GMO (genetically modified organism) is the result of a laboratory process where genes from the DNA of one species are extracted and forced into the genes of an unrelated plant or animal. This process is called genetic engineering. These foreign genes can come from bacteria, viruses, insects, or animals. They allow crops to be more resistant to pathogens, insects, and pesticides. Herbicide-Tolerant (HT) crops (Roundup Ready® crops) are developed to survive application of a specific herbicide known as Roundup, which previously would have destroyed the crop along with targeted weeds. This provides farmers with a more effective weed control process. Unfortunately, it also means that farmers can use more pesticides, which potentially result to more residues on our produce. In March 2015, the World Health Organization's International Agency for Research on Cancer classified glyphosate, the active chemical in Roundup, as "probably carcinogenic in humans".

https://www.iarc.fr/en/media-centre/iarcnews/pdf/MonographVolume112.pdf

Insect-resistant crops contain the gene from the soil bacterium Bt (Bacillus thuringiensis). These bacteria produce a protein that is toxic to specific insects, providing protection to the plant over its entire life. Nevertheless, the safety of this foreign protein in our bodies is a continued debate among experts.

Common GMO crops in the United States include: corn, soy, cotton, alfalfa, rapeseed (canola), and sugar beet. Currently, up to 92% of U.S. corn is genetically engineered (GE), as are 94% of soybeans and 94% of cotton (cottonseed oil is often used in food products). Much of the corn and soy grown in the United States goes into animal feed, while the remainder is processed into various ingredients, such as high-fructose corn syrup, corn oil and corn starch, soy oil, or used as the raw material to make many other ingredients often found in processed foods. In this way, GMO crops contribute to our highly-processed food diet, by supporting low production costs of these foods.

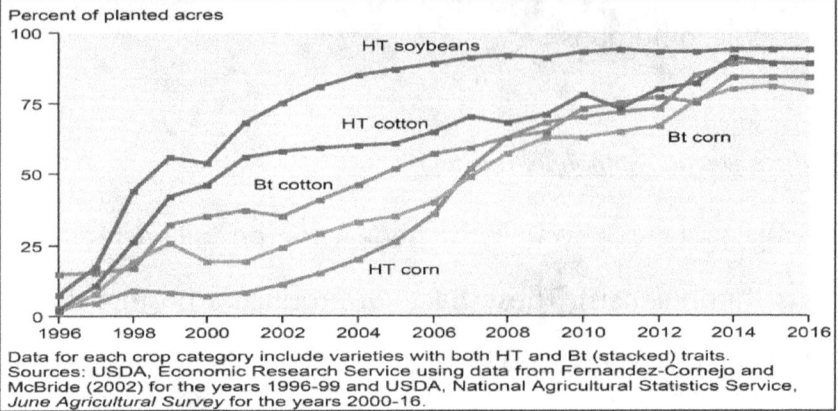

Adoption of genetically engineered crops in the United States, 1996-2016

Percent of planted acres

HT soybeans

HT cotton

Bt corn

Bt cotton

HT corn

Data for each crop category include varieties with both HT and Bt (stacked) traits.
Sources: USDA, Economic Research Service using data from Fernandez-Cornejo and
McBride (2002) for the years 1996-99 and USDA, National Agricultural Statistics Service,
June Agricultural Survey for the years 2000-16.

Figure 6: Evolution of some GMOs crops among USA formers from 1996 to 2016

Source: https://www.ers.usda.gov/data-products/adoption-of-genetically-engineered-crops-in-the-us/recent-trends-in-ge-adoption/

To summarize, we can say that a scientific revolution during World War II, the labor shortage of that time, governmental policies, which subsidized certain foods, and TV ads have all contributed to the proliferation of our fast and highly processed food diet. Further, this has been facilitated by lower, production costs, and the introduction, in 1996, of GMO crops, increasingly found in processed foods. Consequently, we have gone from a society that cooked at home, with whole food ingredients, to one highly reliant on canned and frozen dinners, boxed foods, and fast foods, as a replacement for homemade meals.

Chapter Two
Processed vs. Whole Foods

❖❖❖❖❖❖

*T*he common food of our ancestors was what today we call organic, or whole foods. Unfortunately, these foods have become a luxury for many, considering that ultra-processed foods have become the norm, and tend to be less expensive than non-processed. However, what is the difference between whole food and processed foods?

Whole food is that which has gone through little or no processing. It still contains its natural composition. This natural composition includes: vitamins, minerals, amino acids, fatty acids, carbohydrates, fibers, enzymes, and phytochemicals. Such compounds work together to nourish the body and support health, through proper, immune-response, detoxification and cellular rejuvenation. Ultra-processed foods, on the other hand, have lost much of their natural composition, during the processing procedure. Additionally, ingredients, such as salt, fat, and sugar, are often added in high quantities, as well as other artificial additives meant for other purposes. The rationale is to improve flavor, texture, appearance, and preservation. Sadly, the combination of these added ingredients is known to excite our taste buds, resulting in an addictive cycle, causing one to desire to increase consumption. As we know, more food means more calories, which has the potential of leading to obesity and its related conditions, such as heart disease and certain types of cancer.

An example, of how highly processed and fast foods can affect our health, is highlighted in the documentary, *"Supersize Me"*, released in 2004. In this expose, Morgan Spurlock decided to eat all of his meals at McDonald's, for a month. For 30 days, he would take breakfast, lunch, and dinner at McDonald's, including fountain drinks. As the film progresses, you see Spurlock's physical and emotional health begin to deteriorate, because of this fast food diet. First, he began to feel unusually tired, followed by headaches, and a sense of increasing depression and anxiety each day. He developed an addiction for the fast food, causing him to want greater and greater quantities. His liver began to fill up with fat, from the high level of fat and sugar in his diet. His blood sugar and cholesterol rose abruptly, and his blood pressure became uncontrollably high.

At this point, Spurlock's doctors and family urged him to stop this destructive experiment, but he was determined to complete the thirty days. The result was a weight gain of 24.5 lbs. and a deplorable state of health. Spurlock's girlfriend, a vegan chef, took on the project to detox him, by placing him on a whole food plant-based diet, to restore balance to his body. After six weeks of this regimen, his cholesterol and liver functions returned to normal, and his overall health drastically improved.

This documentary is an unexpected eye-opener for viewers, and clearly demonstrates how a fast food diet can quickly impact one's health in a negative manner. Though some might argue that it is not common for a person to be so extreme, as to eat fast food three times a day, the reality is that there are many people who do eat this way on a regular basis. In any case, the film clearly shows that a fast food diet can have a major, negative impact on the quality of one's health. Its deterioration can be abrupt or at a slower rate, depending on how much one consumes. The film also shows the power of whole food plant-based diet to heal the body. It demonstrates that Spurlock began to feel better, within a very short time on this diet.

Like most Americans, you probably grew up on the Standard American Diet, where ultra-processed and fast foods were the staple—not realizing the impact they have on weight and overall health. The picture below shows a sample breakfast, from a fast food restaurant. Note the outrageous number of calories, fat, and sodium that would be consumed.

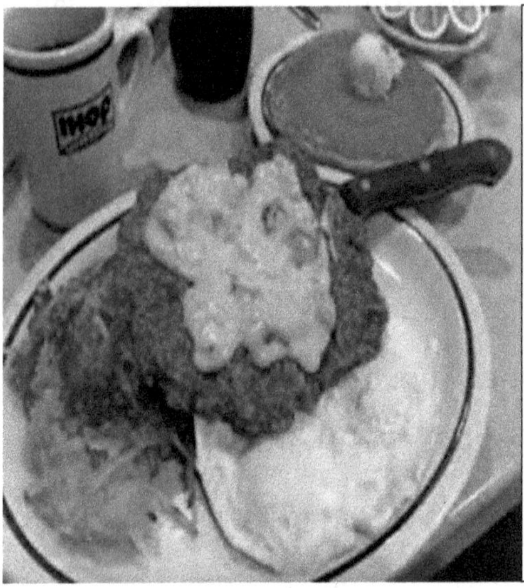

Cal:	2,510
Total fat:	163 g
Saturated fat:	54 g
Trans fat:	3 g
Cholesterol:	800 mg

Figure 7: Chicken/Country Fried Steak & Eggs w/Sausage Gravy from Ihop

Source: Company website

Fast food meals are often high in calorie, fat, sodium, and sugar. Let's take a quick look at each of these elements:

- Calories

A calorie is a unit of energy that is essential to one's good health. It is for the body what gas is to the car. The number of calories on nutritional labels shows just how much energy is derived from a particular food. The key is to take in the right amount for your body. Numbers vary from person to person, depending on factors, such as age, sex, size, and level of activity. The common recommendation for an average man is 2,500 calories per day and 2,000 calories per day for an average woman. Unfortunately, it is very easy to exceed this daily recommendation with just from one meal. The consequence is that calories are stored in the body as fat, which then leads to obesity. For this reason, more than one-third (36.5%) of U.S. adults are struggling with obesity.

http://www.cdc.gov/obesity/data/adult.html

- Fat

Despite what one might think, fat is needed by the body for many functions including the absorption of vitamin A, D, K, and E. It also cushions our vital organs, helps maintain our core temperature, and supports the production of hormones. Nevertheless, it should be good fats and in moderation. Most fast foods are high in saturated fat, from an animal source, as well as trans-fatty acids, from deep frying. Processed foods also often contain partially hydrogenated soy bean oil. This process of hydrogenation forms trans-fatty acids, and excessive consumption of these fats has been linked to plaque buildup in the arteries and heart diseases.

Our pictured Chicken/Country Fried Steak & Eggs w/Sausage Gravy, from Ihop, has 54 g of saturated fat and 3 g of trans-fat. The Dietary Guidelines for Americans, in 2015, recommends limiting saturated fat to no more than 20 grams a day, and avoidance of trans-fat. It is, therefore, shocking to see how one meal alone can exceed these recommendations. This explains why approximately 85.6 million Americans are living with some form of cardiovascular disease, or the after-effects of a stroke.

http://www.onebraveidea.com/submissions/ucm_470704.pdf

- Sodium

Sodium (salt) is also an essential nutrient needed by the body, but in a relatively small amount. It works along-side potassium and magnesium to regulate blood pressure. However, consuming too much sodium often tends to increase blood pressure, putting one at risk of cardiovascular disease, congestive heart failure, and kidney disease. Studies have shown that a majority of the USA population consumes much more sodium than needed, averaging 3,400 mg a day. The recommendation is for no more than 2,300 mg (one teaspoon) a day and less than 1,500 mg a day for certain people. Processed and fast foods are typically high in sodium, as it is also used as a preservative.

Our Chicken/Country Fried Steak example has a sodium content of 5,450 mg. This is more than three days' worth of sodium, for someone who is 65 or over, or someone who has diabetes, high blood pressure, or is African American. The recommendation for these groups of people is, no more than 1,500 mg of sodium per day. Additionally, one third of the population has a pre-hypertensive condition that increases the risk of developing high blood pressure. Nearly 80 million people are diagnosed with it, and almost 75% of those are using anti-hypertensive medication—only 52% who's condition is under control.

https://www.heart.org/idc/groups/heart-public/@wcm/@sop/@smd/documents/downloadable/ucm_319587.pdf

- Added Sugar

Sugar is naturally found in wholefoods, but much, of the sugar in our diet today, is added during processing. It is added to most processed food, usually, in the form of high fructose corn syrup, and is found in high amounts, even in savory food. Food manufacturers frequently use high fructose, corn syrup for viscosity (thickening), texture, enhancement of the browning process, as well as preservation. To cover up for this excess of sugar, they add more salt. This explains why processed foods are typically high in both sugar and salt. The American Heart Association (AHA) suggests limiting the amount of added sugars to no more than 6 teaspoons (24 grams) of sugar per day for women, and 9 teaspoons (36 grams) of sugar per day for men. The Dietary Guidelines for Americans recommends that we should keep our intake of added sugars to less than 10% of total daily calories. For example, in a 2,000 daily calorie diet no more than 200 calories should come from added sugars. The average American consume 22 teaspoons of added sugar per day, corresponding to 88 grams and 352 calories; considering there are 4 grams of sugar in one teaspoon, and 4 calories in one gram of sugar. Obviously if you are on the standard american diet, it is almost impossible to meet these recommendations due to the high intake of sugary beverages, snacks and sweets.

The graph below shows the common source of excess sugar in our diet. As you can see, fruits and vegetables contribute only 1% each, and grains only 8%. Drinks, snacks and sweets contribute to the majority of the added sugar consumed.

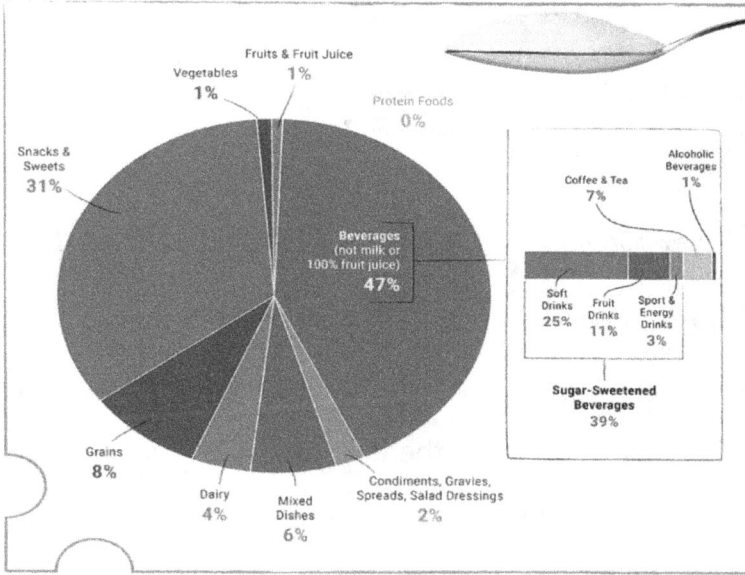

Figure 8: Source of sugar in the American Standard diet

Source: Diatery Guidelines for Americans 2015

High quantities of refined sugar create a spike in blood sugar levels, leading to insulin resistance, which then contributes to obesity and Type 2 diabetes. The result is that 29.1 million people have Type 2 diabetes and 86 million people are pre-diabetic, a condition that puts you at risk of developing the condition.

http://www.cdc.gov/diabetes/data/statistics/2014statisticsreport.html

- **Food additives**

Food additives are generally found in fast and processed foods as preservatives, food coloring agents, and taste enhancers.

According to the Environmental Working Group (EWGs), more than 10,000 additives are allowed in food, and the safety of most has not been established.

http://www.ewg.org/research/ewg-s-dirty-dozen-guide-food-additives

Many of these chemicals have recently raised concerns as being linked to serious health problems, including endocrine disruption and cancer. Nevertheless, there is ongoing debate about the effects of the synthetic FD&C colors, such as blue #1 and #2, yellow #5 and #6, and red #40, on conditions, such as asthma, allergies, and eczema, as well as behavior of children.

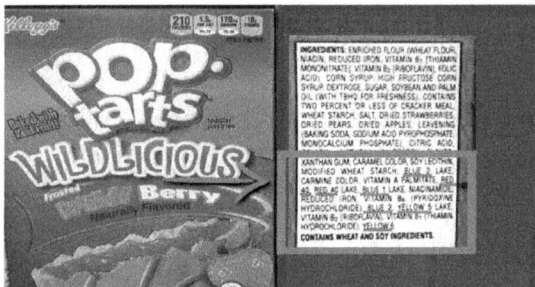

Source: *http://althealthworks.com/8860/americans-eat-5x-more-food-dye-today-causing-horrible-damage-to-kids-healthyelena/*

It is unfortunate that much of the food and drinks, advertised to attract children, contain these food dyes, and may explain the increasing rate of ADHD and asthma seen in children. Such artificial food dyes are banned in Norway and Austria, and the

European Union requires a warning notice placed on most foods containing them— *"Consumption may have an adverse effect on activities and attention in children"*.

Fortunately, the Center for Science in the Public Interest (CSPI) has released a report that there is a potential for artificial food dyes to contribute to hyperactivity in children, an increase in cancer risk, and an adverse effect health issues. The full PDF document is linked below.

https://cspinet.org/new/pdf/food-dyes-rainbow-of-risks.pdf

Food colorings, as mentioned, are still allowed in the United States, and without any warnings. The FDA currently holds the position that they have not found any conclusive evidence that food dyes cause behavior problems in children, but that some children may be susceptible, or prone to, increased symptoms of ADHD, with the consumption of these dyes. They state:

"Exposure to food and food components, including artificial food colors and preservatives (AFC), may be associated with adverse behaviors, not necessarily related to hyperactivity, in certain susceptible children with ADHD and other problem behaviors, and possibly in susceptible children from the general population".

Synthetic food dye, however, is just one example of controversial, food additives in our diet. Other questionable ingredients include: propyl gallate, used as a preservative in products that contain edible fats found in sausage; propyl paraben, added as a preservative in tortillas, muffins; as well as potassium bromate, employed to bolster bread and cracker dough, during the rising process, prior to baking. Nitrites and nitrates are also used as preservatives in cured meats, such as bacon, salami, sausages and hot dogs. Additionally, BHT (butylated hydroxytoluene) is often identified in boxed cereals, as well as BHA (butylated hydroxyanisole), added to chips and preserved meat. Sadly, these types of food additives are being linked to such health issues as cancer. Some have even been classified as endocrine-disroptors.

As is evident, the danger of a diet primarily based on fast and processed foods is no longer in question. Many studies have established the link between certain common ingredients in these foods and most of the health issues affecting us today. Sadly, an analysis, of the grocery purchases in the United States, reveals that more than 60% of the calories we take in are from highly processed foods.

Thusly, as already mentioned, ultra-processed foods are being depleted of most substances that nourish the body and loaded with potentially harmful ingredients. This practice leaves the body increasingly vulnerable to decay and disease. No wonder why the rate of chronic and degenerative disease is so high today.

The strategy, therefore, must be to find ways to consume more whole foods, in order to boost nutrients intake. By doing so we will be providing the body with the proper tools to protect itself from those degenerative diseases, and to support healing.

NOTES

Chapter Three
Reclaiming Your Health

❖❖❖❖❖❖

S uccess in controlling the spread of infectious diseases is primarily attributable to the progress that science continues to make in developing, and introducing, new vaccines and antibiotics. However, when it comes to chronic (ongoing) disease, medications are often merely used to manage symptoms, rather than cure the illnesses themselves. Despite new medical procedures and medications, almost half of all adults in the USA still suffer from one or more chronic health conditions today.

http://www.cdc.gov/chronicdisease/overview/

Pills are not the only answer, however, to the health crisis of this generation. We have eaten our way into this problem, and the best way to combat it is to eat our way out—this plus other life-style changes. The World Health Organization has concluded that eating nutritious foods, becoming more physically active, and avoiding tobacco can help keep us from developing many of our foremost, chronic conditions. For instances, simple lifestyle changes of this type can potentially prevent 80% of heart disease and stroke, 80% of Type 2 diabetes, and 40% of cancer. The good news is that, even if one is already diagnosed with one of these chronic conditions, developing healthy life-style habits can go a long way toward better managing an illness, avoid complications, promote healing, and prolong life.

http://www.who.int/chp/chronicdiseasereport/part1/en/index11.html

The fact that these percentages are so high is good news. Should health conditions run in a family, it doesn't mean there is nothing that can be done, or that they are inevitable. The problem today is that, rather than working diligently to modify diets and lifestyle habits, to effectively prevent or eventually reverse chronic disease, many people prefer the easier option of taking pills to control their chronic symptoms. Furthermore, it is convenient to blame the government for food regulations that do not protect consumers, as well as the food industry for making foods that do not support good health.

Although some changes by these two entities could help us improve our diets, we alone are responsible for our choices. At the end of the day, we are all accountable for the care of our own bodies. If we are not in charge of the foods we eat, then our food is in charge of us. Sadly, for most of us, our food is controlling us to death.

According to the Centers for Disease Control and Prevention (CDC), chronic diseases and conditions—such as heart disease, stroke, cancer, type 2 diabetes, obesity, and arthritis—are among the most common, costly, and preventable of all health problems.

In our nation, chronic diseases account for most health care cost, and are also the main cause of disability. For instance Diabetes is currently the leading cause of kidney failure, lower-limb amputations (other than those caused by injury), and new cases of blindness among adults. The total estimate of diagnosed diabetes in 2012 was $245 billion. Total annual cardiovascular disease costs to the nation averaged $316.1 billion in 2012–2013. Cancer care cost $157 billion in 2010, and, in 2008, medical costs linked to obesity were estimated to be $147 billion. The total cost of arthritis and related conditions was about $128 billion in 2003. Also arthritis is repported to be the most common cause of disability.

Imagine the quality of life possible, without symptoms of chronic health conditions, and how much money could be saved on medical bills, if they were prevented from ever developing, all by engaging in some simple life changes.

We live in a fast-paced society, where we want everything readily accessible to us.   Everyone seems to always be in a hurry. Consequently, we consume large quantities of coffee and energy drinks to speed us up, and eat fast foods to save us time. Unfortunately, we don't stop to think that these choices are shortening our lives. A healthy path to regaining our health and extending our lives is to slow down, take time to cook, and enjoy healthy meals.

Many people are confused about what a healthy meal really is, because we are constantly bombarded with mouth-watering images of unhealthy foods in magazines and on TV. A healthy meal is one prepared using a variety of whole plant foods as basic ingredients. Whole food is any kind of food that comes directly from nature, with none or minimal processing. Examples include: fruits, vegetables, whole grains, legumes, nuts, seeds, herbs, spices, and unaltered meats. Minimally processed foods include:

dry herbs and spices, diced tomatoes, tomatoes paste, BPA free canned beans, frozen fruits and vegetables, without any dubious additives.

People often say that it is more expensive to prepare meals at home, using whole food, than it is to buy them from a fast food restaurant. While it is undeniable that acquiring fresh produce can be more challenging, for many people, the exorbitant cost of healthcare to manage chronic diseases, is ultimately more expensive in the long run —accounting for 86% of our nation's health care costs ($2.9 trillion in 2013).

http://www.cdc.gov/chronicdisease/resources/publications/aag/pdf/2015/nccdphp-aag.pdf

By cooking our own food, we have complete control over what we intake. For instance, sodium is a major culprit, when it comes to high blood pressure. As mentioned previously, a diet based on fast and processed foods is unusually high in sodium. It is estimated that reducing the average amount of salt, consumed, from 3,400 mg to 2,300 mg per day, cases of high blood pressure could be reduced by 11 million, while saving $18 billion on health care every year. This is pretty impressive!

http://www.cdc.gov/bloodpressure/facts.htm.

As the link between eating a diet of highly processed foods and contracting degenerative chronic disease has been established, a whole foods plant-based diet obviously makes sense. The best way to achieve this goal is by cooking more meals at home. Although it might appear to be spending more money, in the short run, you may end up prolonging your life and spending less for medical care over a lifetime. Grave complications, a poor quality of life, and thousands of dollars spent on medications are only a few of the problems faced once a disease is diagnosed. To reclaim your health, it is crucial to redefine priorities. Many of us want the nice things of life, and there is nothing wrong with that. However, if choices are detrimental to one's health, there is a major problem. Good health is a crucial asset, and investing in it must be a high priority. When it comes to your health, diet and lifestyle can either fight for you, or against you. The choice is all yours to make. Choose life!

Chapter Four

Nature's "Miracle Pills"

❖❖❖❖❖❖

*H*ippocrates, the Father of modern medicine, said centuries ago, *"Let thy food be thy medicine and thy medicine be thy food."*

In Hippocrates day, they didn't have ultra-processed or fast food, but I am certain that he was referring to real, or whole foods, taken from nature—the food that God intended from the beginning, for us to eat. Following the creation of the first man and first woman (Adam Eve), God gave them directions about what to eat. He said, *"See, I have given you every herb that yields seed, which is on the face of all the earth, and every tree whose fruit yields seed; to you it shall be for food"* (Gen. 1:29*).*

From this scripture, the original plan for mankind was to have a variety of fruits, seeds, nuts, and vegetables as a major part of their diet. Following the fall of Adam and Eve, God gave them further instructions about their diet. *"Every moving thing that lives shall be food for you. I have given you all things, even as the green herbs. But you shall not eat flesh with its life, that is, its blood"* (Gen. 9:3-4). Although the Bible does not say there is anything wrong with eating meat, much research shows that a plant-based diet is by far best for one's health. Thusly, when you realize that plant foods were what God originally recommended, it validates this conclusion.

Many studies have revealed that cultures that rely on a whole food plant-based diet, of fruits, vegetables, whole grains, legumes, nuts, and seeds have a reduced rate of many preventable diseases common in western societies—illnesses, such as heart disease, cancer, and Type 2 diabetes. This type of diet is highly acclaimed by health experts, for its provable health benefits. A plant-based diet, however, does not have to be a vegetarian diet. Meat can be included; just in smaller quantities, as compared to what people is being consumed today. *The Dietary Guidelines for American 2015* recommend that meat should cover no more than one-quarter of a plate. In the typical American meal, meat occupies the largest part of the plate, which contributes to excess calories with a high fat content. Obviously, that leaves less room for more nutritious food groups, such as vegetables.

As mentioned in previous chapters, calories are to the body, as fuel is to the car, or engine. They are required for the body to function efficiently. Macronutrients are carbohydrates, proteins, and fat—the basic components of every diet, and contain measurable calories. One gram of carbohydrates provides 4 calories, and one gram of protein 4 calories. One gram of fat, however, has a calorie count of 9 calories. Therefore, a diet high in meat is also high in calories—especially when consuming conventionally raised meat; it contains more fat than pasture raised meat. Therefore, the challenge is to maintain a balance in macronutrients, without consuming more than is needed.

Just like the car, however, the body requires more than gas alone. For instance, without the right type of oil in appropriate quantities, a car will not run efficiently. Even if it is working well today, if simple maintenance is ignored, the engine can be damaged, and the car need repair. The same is true of the body. Unless it is maintained adequately, unnecessary damage can occur, leading to preventable consequences.

Originally, the benefits of plant foods were attributed to the abundance of micronutrients, or vitamins and minerals. Recent research studies, however, demonstrate that thousands of other compounds also hold the keys to good health. These compounds are called phytochemicals, AKA phytonutrients. 'Phyto' means plant, thus phytochemicals are 'plant chemicals.'

Phytochemicals are naturally occurring, biologically active chemical compounds in plants that have protective and disease preventive properties. Plants produce these chemicals to protect themselves against UV ray damage, air pollutants, oxidation, bacteria, fungi, and insects. Recent research studies, however, show that they can also protect the human body against certain diseases and damage. There are thousands of phytochemicals providing different benefits, such as antioxidant, anti-inflammatory, and detoxification support. Considering that most chronic diseases affecting us today are linked to the oxidative damage caused by free radicals, chronic inflammation, and poor detoxification, increasing the intake of phytochemicals is a positive way to prevent these conditions. Furthermore, it has been established that the same nutrients that prevent the initial development of diseases can also halt, or reverse them, once diagnosed.

In his book *Eat to Live*, Dr. Joel Fuhrman emphasizes the benefit of phytochemicals to the body's health. He contends that:

"When we consume a sufficient variety and quantity of phytochemical substances, to maximally arm our immune defenses against cancer, we afford ourselves the ability to repair DNA damage, detoxify cancer-causing agents, and resist disease in general."

He refers to phytonutrients as Nature's 'Magic Pills'. Phytochemicals, therefore, along with vitamins and minerals are like the oil that keeps an engine running smoothly. By comparison, good health and longevity rely heavily on the adequate amount and variety of these 'Magic Pills'.

When it comes to improving the American diet, the nutrients most lacking are phytochemicals. For instances, research suggests that to lower the risk of cancer and other chronic diseases, what is missing from our diet is even more important than what is in it. Thusly, to reclaim good health, emphasis must be placed on increasing the intake of such phytochemical elements as vitamins and minerals. Though their absence from the diet might not cause deficiency symptoms, research studies indicate that phytochemicals may reduce the risk of many chronic diseases like cancer, Type 2 diabetes, and heart disease. These findings are interesting, considering how much money is spent by the public, on multivitamins and mineral supplements, and yet there is still no improvement in chronic disease statistics. More than one-third of all Americans take multivitamin/mineral (MVM) supplements. Sales of all dietary supplements in the United States were estimated at $36.7 billion in 2014. Although they might be helpful in some cases, it is obvious that they are not as effective in preventing chronic diseases or addressing the deficiency of phytonutrients in today's diet. *https://ods.od.nih.gov/factsheets/Mvms-HealthProfessional/*

Have you ever heard someone say, "My cholesterol and blood pressure were high and my blood sugar unmanageable, but when I started taking multivitamin/mineral supplements everything went back to normal?" Probably not! However, I have seen people struggling with Type 2 diabetes, high cholesterol, and high blood pressure that were out of control, even with medication. When the diet was changed, by consuming more leafy vegetables, fruits, and nuts, however, the result was incredible. Looking again at Morgan Spurlock's documentary *Supersize Me,* in which he described the devastating effects of his MacDonald experiment, we saw weight gain, non-alcoholic fatty liver disease, high blood pressure, elevated blood sugar, and heightened cholesterol. Nevertheless, he shared how his body came back into balance after only six weeks of following a plant-based diet. That's the power of phytochemicals!

If you want to experience the benefits of these amazing compounds, you must make certain to include a variety of colorful fruits and vegetables in your diet, as they are high in phytochemicals. Other plant foods, such as whole grains, legumes, nuts, seed, herbs, and spices are also excellent sources of phytonutrients. These same foods are also high in vitamins and minerals. Even though many people take vitamin and mineral supplements, nothing can replace the synergistic effect of the nutrients in whole foods.

Although all plant foods contain nutrients, not all of them are equal in content or value. When it comes to preventing diseases, or healing the body with foods, selection must target the ones that provide the highest quantity and variety of nutrients. If, like most Americans, the potato is your primary vegetable, and orange juice your first source of fruit, you probably won't experience the full benefit of a plant-based diet. It is necessary to consume foods with the highest amount and variety of phytonutrients. Studies have shown that these compounds are most abundant in colored fruits and vegetables, including berries and leafy green vegetables. Unfortunately, these are the least consumed in our society, as illustrated in the charts below.

Most commonly consumed vegetables among U.S. consumers, 2014

Pounds per person

■ Fresh ▪ Canned ■ Frozen ▪ Dehydrated ■ Potato Chips

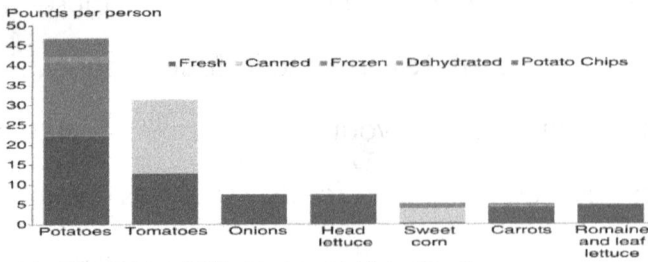

Potatoes Tomatoes Onions Head lettuce Sweet corn Carrots Romaine and leaf lettuce

Loss-adjusted food availability data are proxies for consumption.
Source: USDA, Economic Research Service, Loss-Adjusted Food Availability Data.

Most commonly consumed fruits among U.S. consumers, 2014

Pounds per person

■ Fresh ▪ Canned ■ Frozen ▪ Dried ■ Juice

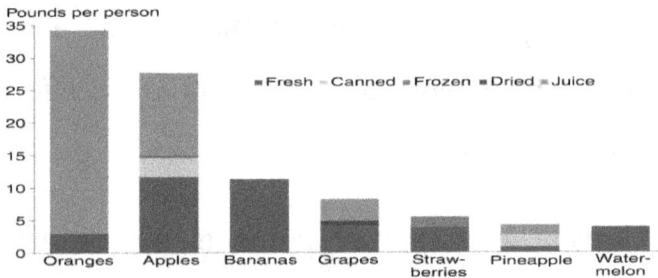

Oranges Apples Bananas Grapes Strawberries Pineapple Watermelon

Loss-adjusted food availability data are proxies for consumption.
Source: USDA, Economic Research Service, Loss-Adjusted Food Availability Data.

Source: *https://www.ers.usda.gov/data-products/ag-and-food-statistics-charting-the-essentials/food-availability-and-consumption/*

In summary, when trying to make healthier food choices, many people feel challenged by the time factor involved in preparing whole foods, as well as the high cost of these food products. We live in a fast-passed society, where time is a rare commodity, and changing eating habits from convenient, fast and processed foods, to more nourishing homemade, meals, is not something that will happen overnight. It will require a re-education about nutrition, some practical incentives, and efforts to lower the cost of healthier foods. In the mean-time, the lack of crucial nutrients, such as phytochemicals needed to prevent disease and support healing, will remain a problem. The challenge is to increase the intake of phytochemicals, in a convenient way that fits into busy lifestyles. This is the motivation for my growing passion to develop 'Superfood' or 'power smoothies' that enhance the nutrient value of dietary consumption. In the next section of this book, the benefits of these smoothies will be discussed, along with their preventive and healing qualities.

NOTES

Chapter Five
If You Can't Eat Them, Drink Them!

❖❖❖❖❖❖

*T*hree years ago, my husband returned from his annual, medical check-up, with a prescription for a statin drug to lower his cholesterol. At that time, I was just beginning my journey toward more healthy living, and learning about the benefits of a plant-based diet. Because taking the prescribed medication was not a life or death matter, we decided to first try to address the cholesterol issue, with a change in diet. I had become aware of incorporating more fruits and vegetables into our diet, through the addition of superfood-smoothies. As I learned how this easy practice could

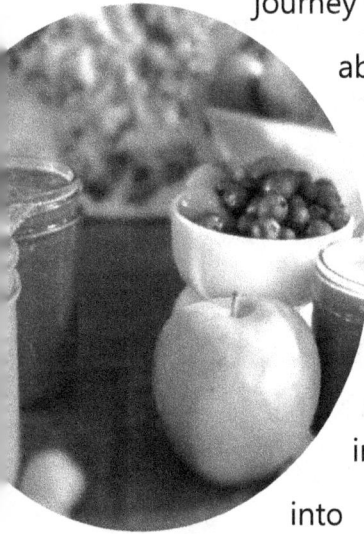

improve overall health, I introduced them to my family. They are, now, a routine part of our diet.

It was a challenge, at first, to get my husband onboard. Because he was determined to improve his health without medication, however, he willingly gave this new regimen a try. He was fighting for his health, so he dedicated himself to this rather novel idea of drinking the foods his body was lacking. To his amazement, it wasn't so bad, and he began to accept whatever superfoods I gave him, in this liquid form.

After three months of drinking superfood-smoothies, at least five days a week, my husband had his cholesterol checked again. Wonder of wonders, his numbers were back to normal. He never took one pill of the prescribed medication. Naturally, we were thrilled by the results, so we decided to make even more changes to our diet. Today, we are convinced of the health benefits of this regimen, as day after day we see an improvement in our overall health. Not only are our health stats improved, but we are more resistant to common colds and viruses. Daily life and family plans are no longer interrupted by typical illnesses that keep us from doing the things we must and would like to do.

An amazing thing about superfood-smoothies is that you can target specific body systems, with a careful selection of superfoods. For example, as I did with my husband's cholesterol issue, it was possible to select superfoods that support the cardiovascular system. During winter, I often select superfoods that support the respiratory and the immune system; and this practice has allowed us to enjoy healthier winters. We used to be very sick with the flu, whether we took the flu shot or not. With superfoods smoothies as part of our diet, even if we catch a cold, the recovery time is way shorter than before.

Through further research, I learned more about the structure, content, and potential of healthy foods in our diet, and my passion for superfood-smoothies was born. This provided an easy, and agreeable, way of incorporating added nutrients into the diet. Excited, I started to share my knowledge with other people, by teaching classes in my home, and later at a local gym and churches. During these classes, the interest and excitement of the attendees, as well as the questions they asked, revealed that there was not enough time to share all that I knew, during these short sessions. That became the motivation for this book. It would allow the 'wholefood message' to be spread more widely, and enable people to take greater control of their own health issues.

I have heard people say they have tried various kinds of vegetable smoothies, but did not like the taste or texture. After sampling options, I prepared in class, however, I would hear, "Wow, that's good!" This would make me smile, because I know there are ways to make smoothies taste better, and encourage people to consume them daily. Taste does matter, and sharing my kitchen-tested tips, to make power-smoothies taste good, is the basis of this book. When you can combine good taste with health benefits, you have created a winning combination.

As mentioned in previous chapters, preventing disease and improving health, is as much about what is missing from a diet as what needs to be cut out. I strongly believe that, if you focus on ways to introduce what is missing, you will automatically diminish the intake of what is unhealthy. We know that phytochemicals are the primary missing compounds, and that they are abundant in plant foods, such as fruits, leafy greens and other colorful vegetables. So, if you have been looking for ways to get on a healthy track, start making superfood-smoothies.

No prior cooking experience is necessary to make a superfood smoothie. A young person can be taught to concoct a healthy drink for a snack, rather than grabbing a coke and bag of chips. Smoothies are a quick and easy way to introduce nourishing food into the diet, without expending a lot of time and money. Many studies have shown that raw fruits and vegetables, especially green leafy vegetables, hold the key to promoting health and preventing diseases. They are what is most missing from today's diet. I am not talking about putting a leaf of iceberg lettuce and a slice of tomato on a hamburger. I am talking about incorporating appropriate quantities of greens and other vegetables, beside potatoes, into the daily diet. The U.S. National Institute of Health (NIH) through the DASH Diet (Dietary Approaches to Stop Hypertension) recommends a daily intake of 8-10 servings of fruit and vegetables per day, as part of dietary changes to prevent and treat high blood pressure. These same recommendations have also been endorsed by many other health and nutrition experts, as an effective tool to healing the body.

How big is a serving?

For vegetables: 1 cup raw, leafy green vegetable = 1 serving

½ cup of any other vegetable, cooked or raw = 1 serving

½ cup vegetable juice = 1 serving

For fruit: 1 med fruit such as an apple, pear, orange, banana, or grapefruit = 1 serving

½ cup fresh or frozen fruit = 1 serving

½ cup fruit juice = 1 serving

¼ cup dry fruit = 1 serving

https://www.nhlbi.nih.gov/files/docs/public/heart/dash brief.pdf

While these recommendations may seem somewhat intimidating at first, by making power-smoothies part of your diet, it is more do-able than you might think. It is a simple and easy way to make certain that you meet the minimum amount of nutrients the body requires to function at its optimum level.

In my journey to increasing the intake of fruits and vegetables, I have also experimented with juicing. I soon learned that both power-smoothies and juicing were powerful tools to boosting the intake of phytochemicals and other nutrients, while improving health.

People often ask me, "What is the difference, from a health standpoint, between juicing and superfood-smoothies?" Keep reading... we will cover that later in this book.

NOTES

Chapter Six
Health Benefits of Superfood-Smoothies

❖❖❖❖❖❖

A Superfood-Smoothie is a highly nutritious, smooth, and relatively thick drink made with a careful selection of fruit, vegetables, and other plant foods known as superfoods. Other common names for these smoothies are 'green smoothies', and 'power-smoothies'. These super- drinks provide many health benefits including:

- ## Intake of more nutrients

By having a daily superfood-smoothie, you automatically increase your intake of raw fruits and vegetables, primarily leafy, green vegetables. They are the ones most missing from the average diet. These foods are not only high in phytochemicals, but also in fiber and a wide range of vitamins and minerals. The Dietary Guidelines for Americans reports that Americans do not consume enough vitamin A, vitamin D, vitamin E, folate, iron, vitamin C, calcium, magnesium, potassium, and fiber—all of which are crucial to maintaining overall good health. For instance, vitamin C acts as an antioxidant, which protects cells from oxidative damage. Potassium and magnesium support a healthy blood pressure, thus promoting cardiovascular health. Unfortunately, most people are taking dietary supplements to compensate for a poor diet. Nevertheless, nothing can replace the synergistic effect of all the nutrients contained in wholefoods.

- **Improved digestion and absorption of nutrients**

Increasing intake of nutrients, by consuming more fruits and vegetables, is one thing; making sure they are absorbed effectively by the body is another. We often hear that digestion starts in the mouth, with the proper mastication (chewing) of our food. Unfortunately, our busy lifestyles tend to cause us to eat too fast. This results in poor digestion, and, consequently, poor absorption of nutrients. In the preparation of a superfood-smoothie, all ingredients are blended together into a tasty, smooth drink, making it much easier for the body to assimilate. Further, as we already know, the standard American diet is deficient in fiber, which also can cause constipation. It is no wonder that laxatives are one of the most frequently purchased over the counter medications in the United States. Better digestion is one of the first benefits people tend to mention as they incorporate this new regimen into their lifestyle.

- Increased intake of fiber

Since dietary fiber is found only in plant foods, the average American significantly falls short of the recommended 25-30 grams of fiber per day—consuming on average only 12 - 17 grams daily. Research has found that an adequate amount of fiber in the diet actually lowers the risk of diabetes, heart diseases, some cancers, and many other degenerative diseases. Therefore, having a daily superfood-smoothie is a great way to reach, and even exceed, these minimum recommendations.

- Increased energy and mental clarity

In addition to improved digestion, an increase in energy is another initial benefit. This is probably due to the wide range, and heightened level, of nutrients provided by these natural supplement drinks. Almost all, of the people I have talked to, have reported that, when drinking a smoothie in the morning for breakfast, they experienced more energy throughout the day. They also felt more mentally focused. Breakfast options that most people select and enjoy, including certain brands of cereal and fast foods, are generally high in processed carbohydrates and sugar; and poor in phytochemicals. Drinking superfood-smoothies give the brain more of the nutrients needed for optimal functioning.

- **A boost to the immune system**

When the body does not receive all the nutritional value needed to function properly, it is more vulnerable to all kinds of chronic, degenerative, and even infectious diseases. It has been confirmed that one way of preventing cancer and heart disease is to increase the amount of fruit and vegetables in your diet. By so doing, you are enabling every bodily system, particularly the immune system, to perform effectively.

- **Support healing and balance**

The body has the innate ability to heal itself. Nevertheless, it must be provided with the proper tools to do so. As already discussed, phytochemicals are plant chemicals, with the ability to prevent and often reverse certain diseases. These powerful compounds, along with the vitamins, minerals, fiber, and enzymes abundant in plant foods are the tools needed to promote healing and restore balance to affected body systems. Considering that superfood-smoothies are rich in all kinds of nutrients and phytochemicals, making them part of your diet provides the body with the means to heal and balance its internal bodily systems.

- Natural weight management

Unfortunately, when the body does not detoxify itself well; excess toxins are stored in fat tissue, making it difficult to lose weight. If, like most people, your diet is mainly based on processed and fast foods, chances are that your body is not detoxifying as it should. This is due to a lack of proper nutrients, in the diet. Also, hormonal imbalances such as too much cortisol, insulin resistance, and low thyroid hormones are common in our society today, and have been linked to weight gain.

There are some superfoods with known health benefits of regulating hormones. Along with other lifestyle changes, adding these superfoods to your smoothies might help restore balance, thus contributing to better weight management. When my clients express a desire to lose weight, we often start with a detox plan based on superfood-smoothies that yield significant results. I have provided that eating plan at the end of this book, to kick-start your weight loss journey, or to just boost your health.

Most weight loss programs are very restrictive, depriving people from the foods they enjoy, and leaving them frustrated. No wonder people often jump from one diet program to another, looking for something easier to follow. I don't believe that God created food just for good health. Food is also for our enjoyment, thus contributing somehow to our overall well-being. So completely depriving yourself from the food you enjoy, without any alternative is not a good way to manage your weight.

The healthy way to lose weight is to gradually change your eating habits, by crowding out the junk with more nourishing foods, in a convenient and delightful way that satisfies you. This is a journey where you need to educate yourself on what really nourish your body, and implement a strategy that will become your new lifestyle. However, while you are working on this, you can start losing weight just by making superfood-smoothies part of your diet. You don't have to change anything yet, just take some superfood-smoothie before each main meal (breakfast, lunch, dinner). Doing so will automatically cut down on the amount of food you normally eat, which also means less calories considering that most meals on the American standard way of eating are very high in calories as we learned in previous chapters.

For instance, if you often eat three donuts for breakfast, by drinking some smoothies before your breakfast, you will automatically eat less, probably only one donut. As you know, donut comes with more calories and less nutrients. Smoothie on the other hand comes with fewer calories, and a variety of nutrients and phytochemicals that nourish the body and promote good health. So at the end, you still enjoy your donut, yet you also give your body the nutrient it needs. Losing weight this way is more effective and sustainable. You don't even think about it. Also as you start replacing your poor quality meals and snacks with more nourishing whole foods, you will continue losing even more weight until you reach your healthy level. This is done progressively, without the frustration and guilt that comes with most diet programs.

If you would like to take this journey, but you are not sure where to start, don't worry. We've got you covered. A reset-plan is provided at the end of this book to kick-start weight loss, and boost your health. Remember, this plan is not something to carry on the long run; it is just giving you a place to start. After the 10 days if you need help establishing a healthy lifestyle that support weight loss, contact me for a customized strategy.

Decreased cravings for "junk foods"

As discussed earlier, the combination of common ingredients, such as fat, sugar, salt, and food additives found in processed and fast foods, is designed to stimulate the appetite. Thusly, the more you eat such foods, the more you crave them. Studies have shown that increasing the amount of fruit and vegetables, in your diet, naturally decreases the cravings for 'junk food'. Having a daily, superfood-smoothie is a great way to reduce this condition and reach your goal. Moreover, superfood-smoothies are high in fiber, and can be high in protein, if added to the drink. This combination prevents blood sugar from spiking, and keeps you feeling full for a longer period. It also decreases a desire to snack.

Healthy "fast food"

With some preparation ahead of time, making a Superfood-smoothie can take less than one minute, and can be taken on-the-go. Here is a go-to, healthy, fast option, loaded with nutrients, yet containing fewer calories than regular fast food.

Chapter Seven
Leafy Greens and Other Vegetables

❖❖❖❖❖❖

*A*lthough any vegetable can be used to make a superfood-smoothie, the most vital vegetables are the leafy green ones. This is due to their richness in nutrients and disease fighting phytochemicals. They also contain the least number of calories, when compared to other vegetables.

Leafy green vegetables used in superfood-smoothies

- Kale

When most people hear the words "green smoothie," what first comes to mind is kale. Due to its incredibly high nutrition profile, this cruciferous vegetable has recently become popular and is recognized as one of the healthiest vegetables being consumed.

Kale provides a wide range of disease-fighting phytochemicals, vitamins and minerals, while being high in protein and fiber. Researchers have identified over 45 different flavonoids in kale, combining both antioxidant and anti-inflammatory benefits. Flavonoids are part of the polyphenol class of phytochemicals, highly praised for their numerous health benefits. Compared to other greens, kale is also high in vitamins K, A, and C. One cup of raw kale provides more than 650% DV (Daily Value) of vitamin K, 200% DV of vitamin A, and over 130% DV of vitamin C. It contains a variety of B vitamins, and is rich in other nutrients, such as manganese, copper, potassium, magnesium, and calcium. The nutrition profile of kale is incredible, which explains its value in any diet. Detoxification at different levels—neutralizing toxins and removing them from the body—cancer prevention, proper immune response, cardiovascular health, healthy vision, and cholesterol lowering capabilities are just a few of its benefits.

Additionally, high amounts of potassium, magnesium, and calcium make kale a crucial vegetable, for people dealing with high blood pressure. These nutrients support healthy blood pressure, by relaxing the blood vessel walls. Moreover, kale is an excellent food choice for weight control. The variety of B-vitamins and high level of iron support a healthy metabolism. One of the primary functions of B-complex is aiding in metabolism of carbohydrates, fats, and proteins. It also assists the body in unlocking and utilizing the energy stored in food. B-complex facilitates the production of L-carnitine—an amino acid that promotes fat burning. Concurrently, iron, as part of the hemoglobin molecule, carries oxygen to the muscles that enables them to exercise and burn fat. The detoxification capacity of kale also enhances the weight loss process.

Taste: strong, semi-bitter

Texture: fibrous and tough.

Blends well with: spinach to offset the bitterness. For beginners, start with baby kale, for it has a milder taste. You can work your way up to curly kale; lacinato kale (darker leaves) should be last, as it has the strongest taste. Many grocery stores offer boxed baby kale mixed with spinach, making it a good place to start.

Key nutrients in kale, with a DV of 4%, or above:

1 cup or 67 grams, raw

Calories: 33   Protein: 2 grams   Fiber: 1 gram

Nutrient	Amount	% of Daily Value (DV)
Vitamin K	547 mcg	684%
Vitamin A	10302 IU	206%
Vitamin C	80.4 mg	134%

Vitamin B6	0.2 mg	9%
Thiamine	0.1 mg	5%
Riboflavin	0.1 mg	5%
Folate	19.4 mcg	5%
Manganese	0.5 mg	26%
Copper	0.2 mg	10%
Calcium	90.5 mg	9%
Iron	1.1 mg	6%
magnesium	22.8 mg	6%
Potassium	299 mg	9%
Phosphorous	37.5 mg	4%

- Spinach

Spinach is loaded with a variety of phytonutrients, and contains more than a dozen different flavonoids, functioning as anti-inflammatory compounds. Besides supplying high levels of antioxidants and anti-inflammatory compounds, it also offers impressive amounts of vitamins and minerals overall, with very few calories. One cup of raw spinach contains only 7 calories, making it also an ideal food for those wishing to lose weight. When considering the nutrition profile of spinach, it is evident that it too is one of the healthiest foods to include in a diet. Among its multiple health benefits, spinach promotes good vision, through carotenoids, lutein, and zeaxanthin. Carotenoids are primary antioxidants in several regions of the eye, including the retina and macula. Abundant levels of antioxidants, in the form of vitamin A and vitamin C, are especially useful in maintaining a strong immune system. The high percentage of vitamin K in spinach helps to regulate the body's inflammatory response, as well as promoting healthy bone growth. It is rich in folate, which is also a vital nutrient for pregnant women, because it plays a critical role in fetal development. Folate is important in DNA synthesis and repair, and essential to the preservation of red blood cells. It is also required for proper brain function—a balanced mental and emotional wellbeing.

Taste: mild and pleasant

Texture: Very soft

Blends well with: any other leafy green vegetable

Key nutrients in spinach, with a DV of 4% or above:

1 cup or 30 grams, raw

Calories: 7   Protein: 1 gram   Fiber: 1 gram

Nutrient	Amount	% of Daily value (DV)
Vitamin K	145 mcg	181%
Vitamin A	2813 IU	56%
Vitamin C	8.4 m	14%
Folate	58.2 mcg	15%
Manganese	0.3 mg	13%
Magnesium	23.7 mg	6%
Iron	0.8 mg	5%

- Swiss Chard

Swiss chard is high in syringic acid, a flavonoid phytonutrient that has been shown to inhibit the activity of the enzyme alpha-glucosidase. When this enzyme is blocked, fewer carbohydrates are broken down into simple sugars, and blood-sugar levels remain more constant. This makes Swiss chard one of the best foods for people dealing with type 2 diabetes or insulin resistance.

Swiss chard is also good for people with high blood pressure, because of the balancing agents, magnesium and potassium. Added health benefits include: antioxidant and anti-inflammatory properties, along with detoxification support provided by certain specific phytonutrients called betalains (also found in beets). Just like spinach, Swiss chard is loaded with a variety of anti-cancer phytochemicals and a wide range of vitamins and minerals, which when combined, support every bodily system. This is a highly nutritious vegetable to add to any diet.

Taste: mild and pleasant compared to kale

Texture: not as soft as spinach, but tender

Blends well with: any other leafy green

Key nutrients in Swiss chard, with a DV of 4% and above:

1 cup or 36 grams, raw

Calories: 7   Protein: 1 gram   Fiber: 1 gram

Nutrient	Amount	% of Daily value (DV)
Vitamin K	299 mcg	374%
Vitamin A	2202 IU	44%
Vitamin C	10.8 mg	18%
Manganese	0.1 mg	7%
Magnesium	29.2 mg	7%
Iron	0.6 mg	4%
Potassium	136 mg	4%

- ## Collard Greens

Collard greens are a type of cruciferous vegetable, like cabbage, kale, broccoli, cauliflower, Brussel sprouts, mustard greens, arugula, watercress, and Bok choy.

One of the most important components of collard greens, and other cruciferous vegetables, is glutathione (a naturally occurring molecule in the body that is found in every cell).   As an antioxidant, it assists the liver to cleanse and detoxify fat, boosts immune function, fights cancer, and protects the body from toxins. Dr. Mark Hyman refers to glutathione as "the Mother of all antioxidants." In one of his articles, he emphasizes the benefits of glutathione: "It is the most important molecule you need to stay healthy and prevent aging, cancer, heart disease, dementia and more, and necessary to treat everything from autism to Alzheimer's disease." Glutathione has also been proven to be successful in the treatment of digestive disorders, such as IBS. These benefits make collard greens and other cruciferous vegetables vital to health.

Taste: stronger than spinach, but less bitter than kale.

Texture: sturdy

Blends well with: mild taste vegetable like spinach and Swiss chard to offset the strong taste

Key nutrients in collard greens, with a DV of 4% and above:

1 cup or 36 grams, raw

Calories: 11   Protein: 1 gram   Fiber: 1 gram

Nutrient	Amount	% of Daily value (DV)
Vitamin K	184 mcg	230%
Vitamin A	2400 IU	48%
Vitamin C	12.7 mg	21%
Vitamin E (Alpha Tocopherol)	0.8 mg	4%
Folate	59.8 mcg	15%
Calcium	52.2 mg	5%
Manganese	0.1 mg	5%

- **Beet Greens**

Often, when purchasing beets, it is likely to find them still attached to their colorful, leafy greens. It is important, however, not to cut them off and discard them. Both beets and their leaves are nutrient powerhouses, with a variety of phytonutrients. They work together to support the cardiovascular system, boost the immune system, detoxify the body, and provide anti-cancer benefits. If you have high blood pressure, both beets and beet greens are important vegetables to include into your diet. Rich in magnesium, potassium, and calcium, this amazing vegetable, helps regulate blood pressure, by relaxing the walls of blood vessels.

If taking a diuretic for high blood pressure, such as hydrochlorothiazide (Esidrix, HydroDiuril), you will benefit from the high potassium level in beet greens. These drugs cause the body to lose potassium, through the elimination of urine, thereby lowering the body's potassium levels. Normal levels are important, for the conduction of electrical signals in the nervous system and heart, preventing an irregular heartbeat.

Taste: very similar to Swiss chard and spinach

Texture: Soft, mellow

Blends well with: any other green vegetable

Key nutrients in beet greens, with a DV of 4% and above:

1 cup or 38 grams, raw

Calories: 8   Protein: 1 gram   Fiber: 1 gram

Nutrient	Amount	% of daily value (DV)
Vitamin K	152 mcg	190%

Vitamin A	2404 IU	48%
Vitamin C	11.4 mg	19%
Riboflavin	0.1 mg	5%
Iron	1.0 mg	4%
Calcium	44.5 mg	4%
Potassium	290 mg	8%
Magnesium	26.mg	7%
Manganese	0.1 mg	7%
Copper	0.1 mg	4%

- **Bok Choy**

Known as Chinese cabbage, Bok choy is a staple vegetable in Chinese cuisine. However, today it is becoming increasingly popular in our society, and is much more widely available, due to its nutritional profile. As part of the cruciferous family, Bok choy provides the same anti-cancer and detoxification benefits as its cousin, collard greens. It too is loaded with phytochemicals and a wide range of nutrients, including vitamins A, C, K, B6, folate, calcium, potassium, and manganese. This nutrition line-up makes Bok choy a great food to include in a power smoothie. It reduces the risk of cancer, supports cardiovascular health, boosts detoxification, and maintains a proper immune response. One of the things people don't like about cruciferous vegetables, however, is their pungent taste. Nevertheless, Bok choy doesn't share this characteristic to the same degree. Its flavor is milder.

Consequently, if you tend to dislike kale, cabbage, collard greens, or mustard greens, Bok choy is a more palatable, cruciferous vegetable.

Taste: distinctive, mild, stronger than spinach, but less than kale and collard greens

Texture: tender

Blends well with: spinach, Swiss chard, & beet greens

Key nutrients in bok choy, with a DV of 4% and above:

1 cup or 38 grams, raw

Calories: 8   Protein: 1 gram   Fiber: 1 gram

Nutrient	Amount	% of daily value (DV)
Vitamin k	31.8 mcg	40%
Vitamin A	3128 IU	63%
Vitamin C	31.5 mg	51%
Vitamin B6	0.1 mg	7%
Folate	46.2 mcg	12%
Calcium	73.5 mg	7%
Potassium	176 mg	5%
Manganese	0.1 mg	6%

- ## Mustard Greens

As a cruciferous vegetable, mustard greens too are loaded with disease-fighting phytonutrients, just like their cousins, collard greens, kale, and Bok choy. Moreover, they provide an impressive list of other nutrients, such as vitamins A, C, K, E, B6, as well as riboflavin, folate, calcium, iron, magnesium, potassium, copper, and manganese. Only 1 cup of raw mustard greens provides more than 100% of the recommended daily amount of vitamin A, and more than 60% of vitamin C. Considering the crucial role these two vitamins play in our immune system, assimilating mustard greens into the diet is a good way to boost resistance to disease.

Nevertheless, despite its incredible nutrients profile, I do not recommend mustard greens for beginners. It would be preferable to try other, milder tasting vegetables, before trying mustard greens. Unfortunately, they are not particularly pleasant tasting, in a smoothie. The first time I tied mustard green, even my smoothie ended up in the trash. Since then, I've learned to make a more acceptable mixture of mustard greens and spinach.

Taste: strong, peppery

Texture: soft

Blends well with: spinach. Start with three parts spinach and one-part mustard green, then you can progress to half and half each.

Key nutrients in mustard greens, with a DV of 4% and above:

1 cup or 56 grams, raw

Calories: 15   Protein: 2 grams   Fiber: 2 grams

Nutrient	Amount	% of Daily Value (DV)

Vitamin K	278 mcg	348%
Vitamin A	5881 IU	118%
Vitamin C	39.2 mg	65%
Vitamin E (Alpha Tocopherol)	1.1 mg	6%
Vitamin B6	0.1 mg	5%
Folate	105 mcg	26%
Riboflavin	01 mg	4%
Calcium	57.7 mg	6%
Iron	0.8 mg	5%
Potassium	198 mg	6%
Magnesium	17.9 mg	4%
Copper	0.1 mg	4%
Manganese	0.3 mg	13%

- ## Turnip Greens

Most people are familiar with turnip root; however, turnip greens are where most of the nutrients are found. Just like other leafy green vegetables, turnip greens offer a storehouse of phytonutrients, vitamins and minerals, and are exceptionally rich in calcium and vitamin E. If you are wanting to increase your intake of these nutrients, turnip greens are an excellent choice. Nutrients in turnip greens boost the body's detox and immune systems, support sound bone health, improve liver function, and fight many diseases, by decreasing free radical damage, and reducing inflammation that's frequently at the root of chronic illnesses.

Although turnip greens offer multiple health advantages, cancer prevention is their primary benefit, because they offer impressive amounts of cancer fighting compounds known as glucosinolate. These molecules provide crucial anti-cancer advantages by facilitating healthy cell production (mitosis) and stimulating cell-death, within cancerous tumors (apoptosis). The glucosinolate levels found in turnip greens are noticeably higher than the quantity found in other leafy greens and cruciferous vegetables. Thusly, if cancer prevention, or treatment, is important to you, turnip greens, along with other cruciferous vegetables, are certainly beneficial to your diet.

Taste: strong, slightly bitter, but less than kale

Texture: sturdy

Blends well with: spinach

Key nutrients in turnip greens, with a DV of 4% and above):

1 cup or 55 grams, raw

Calories: 18   Protein: 1 gram   Fiber: 2 grams

Nutrient	Amount	% of Daily Value (DV)
Vitamin K	138 mcg	173%
Vitamin A	6372 IU	127%

Vitamin C	33.0 mg	55%
Vitamin E (Alpha Tocopherol)	1.6 mg	8%
Vitamin B6	0.1 mg	7%
Folate	107 mcg	27%
Calcium	105 mg	10%
Magnesium	17.1 mg	4%
Potassium	163 mg	5%
Copper	0.2 mg	10%
Manganese	0.3 mg	13%

- Dandelion Greens

To most people's surprise, dandelions contain a powerhouse of nutrients and are commonly known as a medicinal herb, rather than a vegetable. They are one of the best sources of calcium, iron, and many B vitamins, including vitamins B6, B1 (thiamin), and B2 (Riboflavin). Dandelion greens are loaded with phytonutrients, and provide a good source of vitamins A, C, E, and K, as well as the minerals: magnesium, potassium, copper and manganese. Just like other leafy greens, the health benefits of dandelions are numerous. The ability to detoxify the liver, however, is most notable. This alone makes dandelions a vital component to any diet. When the liver functions optimally, it is most effective at cleansing the blood, thus promoting health and vitality. It also helps maintain a healthy weight. Like kale, the variety of B-vitamins, and high level of iron, support healthy metabolism and promote fat burning. Dandelions contribute to healthy bone growth, promote cardiovascular health, and aid in the prevention of cancer, through their antioxidant and anti-inflammatory advantages. Lastly, the elevated amount of vitamin E in dandelions, which is not common in other leafy vegetables, promotes a more youthful looking skin, as well as sustaining healthy hair and scalp.

Note: It is not generally common to find dandelion greens alone, in grocery stores. During spring, however, they can often be found in mixed salads. You can then enjoy them in smoothies, along with the other vegetables in the mix.

Taste: very bitter, much more than kale

Texture: soft

Blends well with: mild tasting greens, preferably spinach

Key nutrients in dandelions, with a DV of 4% and above):

1 cup or 55 grams, raw

Calories: 25   Protein: 1 gram   Fiber: 2 grams

Nutrient	Amount	% of Daily Value (DV)
Vitamin K	428 mcg	535%
Vitamin A	5588 IU	112%
Vitamin C	19.3 mg	32%

Vitamin E (Alpha Tocopherol)	1.9 mg	9%
Vitamin B6	0.1 mg	7%
Thiamin	0.1 mg	7%
Riboflavin	0.1 mg	8%
Folate	14.9 mcg	4%
Calcium	103 mg	10%
Iron	1.7 mg	9%
Magnesium	19.8 mg	5%
Potassium	218 mg	6%
Phosphorus	36.3 mg	4%
Copper	0.1 mg	5%
Manganese	0.2 mg	9%

- **Romaine Lettuce**

Lettuce is generally considered synonymous with salads, but did you know it can also be used in smoothies? Just like other leafy green vegetables, romaine lettuce has a high nutrition profile. It is loaded with antioxidant and anti-inflammatory compounds, as well as vitamins A, C, and K and folate. It is also a good source of other nutrients, such as iron, potassium, magnesium, and manganese. As such, romaine lettuce is a good choice for preventing and/or alleviating many chronic diseases, including cancer, heart disease, Type 2 diabetes, and nervous system disorders. The high levels of vitamins A and C support the immune system, as well as providing antioxidant benefits. Vitamin K regulates normal blood clotting and supports bone health.

Folate is crucial in DNA synthesis and repair, as it encourages cell and tissue growth. Moreover, folate helps metabolize homocysteine into methionine—an essential amino acid. Without adequate folate, homocysteine levels increase, and too much homocysteine has been linked to atherosclerosis and cardiovascular problems. Despite its extremely low-calorie content and high, water volume, romaine lettuce is actually a very nutritious food. However I do not use them in my smoothies. I personally prefer Romaine lettuce as a base for my green salad.

Taste: can be slightly bitter, but nothing like kale or collard greens

Texture: soft

Blends well with: more fibrous greens, that are also mild in taste such as Swiss chard or beet greens.

Key nutrients in romaine lettuce, with a DV of 2% and above—generally likely to use at least 2 cups due to the high, water content:

1 cup or 47 grams, raw and shredded

Calories: 8   Protein: 1 gram   Fiber: 1 gram

Nutrient	Amount	% of Daily Value (DV)
Vitamin A	4094 IU	82%
Vitamin C	11.3	19%
Vitamin K	48.2 mcg	60%

Vitamin B6	-	2%
Folate	63.9 mcg	16%
Thiamine	-	2%
Riboflavin	-	2%
Calcium	15.5 mg	2%
Iron	0.5 mg	3%
Magnesium	6.6 mg	2%
Potassium	116 mg	3%
Manganese	0.1 mg	4%

Summary

When looking at the nutrition profiles of leafy green vegetables, you can readily understand why they are the base of superfood-smoothies. Studies have shown that these are the most nutritious vegetables, with the least number of calories. They are also the ones most lacking in the American diet. They are high in many vitamins and minerals, fiber, and a variety of phytochemicals, including antioxidants and anti-inflammatory compounds. They are also the tools that the body needs for proper detoxification, immune response, repair and regeneration of cells, as well as energy metabolism. Therefore, if you are looking to prevent a disease, alleviate a chronic condition, boost your energy level, or achieve a healthy weight, leafy green vegetables are a wise dietary choice.

Should you live in a region where other leafy greens are available, experiment with them. Just be certain to take into consideration the combination rule, which is based on taste and texture:

Strong tasting greens should be combined with mild tasting greens to offset the strong taste. Greens that are soft and high in water content should be combined with more sturdy and fibrous green to provide some texture to your smoothies.

Other vegetables suitable for smoothies

- Broccoli, Cauliflower, Cabbage, and Brussel Sprouts

Although leafy greens are my favorite for superfood-smoothies, broccoli, Cauliflower, Cabbage, and Brussel sprouts can also be used for smoothies. They are cruciferous vegetables, like kale and collard greens; and for that reason, they offer the same detoxification and anti-cancer benefits. Each provides a wide range of nutrients, and they are all great sources of vitamin C. For instance one cup of raw broccoli provides 110% of DV. Studies show, however, that 50%, or more of vitamin C, may be lost when heated. Because these vegetables are often cooked in some way, and vitamin C is sensitive to high temperatures, adding raw broccoli, or Brussels sprouts, to smoothies, is an excellent way to access the full strength of vitamin C.

- Carrots and Beets

Carrots too are high in vitamin A, with 113% of DV in 1 cup of raw carrot. Ample amounts of antioxidants and other phytonutrients found in this vegetable support heightened, cardiovascular health, vision, detoxification, and cancer prevention.

Beets are a unique source of phytonutrients called betalains, which have been shown to provide antioxidant, anti-inflammatory, and detoxification properties. Betalains are also found in foods like the stems of chard, beet leaves, and rhubarb. These phytonutrients, however, are most concentrated in beets. Should you have a high exposure to toxins, and want to give your body the most detox support possible, consider beets as a part of your diet. When adding them to smoothies, however, they must first be steamed for a smoother texture. The fiber in raw beets is very sturdy and is not necessarily pleasant in smoothies.

Note: When consuming beets, in any measurable quantity, it is possible that your urine may turn pinkish/reddish in color. This condition is known as beeturia, and is estimated to be experienced by 10-15% of adults, consuming beets on a regular basis. While beeturia itself is not considered harmful, it may be a possible indicator of problems with iron metabolism. Individuals, with iron deficiency, iron excess, or specific problems with iron metabolism, are more likely to experience beeturia than individuals with healthy iron metabolism. For this reason, if you notice any symptoms of beeturia, it is recommended that you notify your doctor, and check out possible issues related to your iron status. *https://www.ncbi.nlm.nih.gov/pubmed/8148871*

While beets and carrots can be used in smoothies, they are better suited for juicing, which we will discuss later.

Chapter Eight
What Fruits to Use

❖❖❖❖❖❖

I n previous chapters, we discussed that phytonutrients are disease-fighting compounds, which are abundant in fruits and vegetables. However, not all fruits and vegetables are created equal. Leafy green vegetables and berries provide an incredible amount and variety of phytonutrients. That is why these foods should be considered the "stars" in any smoothie. In the USA, we are blessed to have a wide variety of fruits available year around. Nearly any of our favorites can be found and used in smoothies, at any time of the year. However, berries, such as blueberries, blackberries, raspberries, and strawberries, should play a starring role and be included on a frequent basis.

Common Fruits used in Superfood-Smoothies

- Berries

Berries are rich in nutrients, and have a low glycemic index. This makes them a particularly great fruit choice, for people diagnosed with Type 2 diabetes, or is at a high risk of developing the disease. The glycemic index (GI) is a value assigned to food based on how slowly, or quickly, a food causes an increase in blood glucose levels.

Berries are further recognized for their particularly high content of antioxidants and anti-inflammatory compounds. Studies have shown that chronic inflammation and oxidative damage, at a cellular level, are root causes of many chronic diseases. Consequently, incorporating berries into your diet is a good way to prevent such diseases, or improve conditions already diagnosed.

Blueberries are "superstars" among the berries, in terms of their unique, health benefits. They are ranked as having the highest amount of antioxidant properties among berries available in the USA. They are equally well known for their support of brain fitness and ability to promote healthy blood pressure, by increasing the level of nitric oxide (NO) in the blood. Nitric oxide dilates the blood vessels and helps to maintain their elasticity. In so doing, blood pressure is reduced. If one is, therefore, dealing with elevated blood pressure, or has a family history of Alzheimer's, blueberries in the diet could be extremely beneficial. Additionally, their lipid profile contributes to the reduction of total cholesterol—rising of HDL cholesterol and lowering of triglycerides. Consuming this fruit also prevents the oxidation of LDL cholesterol in the blood vessels, which is linked to plaque build-up and leads to conditions, such as high blood pressure and other cardiovascular diseases.

Cranberries are particularly known for addressing urinary issues, by preventing infection. Many people who suffer from urinary tract infections (UTIs) and find relief from drinking cranberry juice. Researchers have believed, for many years that the acidity of cranberries and cranberry juice, has a healing effect on urinary tract infections. However, more recent research has shown that it's not the acidity in the cranberries, but the presence of certain phytonutrients that are related to the prevention and treatment of UTIs. These phytonutrients act as a barrier to bacteria that might otherwise attack the urinary tract lining.

Cranberries can also prevent stomach ulcers, which are often caused by the growth of a stomach bacteria—Helicobacter pylori. The phytonutrients in cranberries seem to prevent these bacteria from attaching itself to the stomach lining, which is interesting, considering that the infection from H. pylori is very common.

Studies have found that nearly two-thirds of the world's population has it present in their bodies. Uncontrolled stomach ulcers caused by these bacteria, generally cause serious GI discomfort that could potentially lead to stomach cancer. Obviously, including cranberries in the diet would have a significant, positive impact on your general health.

http://www.webmd.com/digestive-disorders/h-pylori-helicobacter-pylori#1

Raspberries provide weight management benefits not found in most other berries. Recent studies suggest that some compounds in raspberries actually increase metabolism in fat cells, thus preventing the storage of excess fat. Raspberries are also high in fiber, with about 8 grams of fiber per cup, while, like many other berries, have a low glycemic index.

Strawberries are exceedingly high in vitamin C, with 113% of the daily value (DV) in just 1 cup. Vitamin C is a crucial nutrient for many functions in the body, including the growth and repair of tissue cells throughout the body. It helps to make collagen—an important protein used to accelerate the growth of skin, cartilage, tendons, ligaments, and blood vessels. Vitamin C also works as an antioxidant, as well as stimulating the immune system to prevent and fight infections like colds and flu. Further, some polyphenols in strawberries aid in the regulation of blood sugar, by inhibiting the activity of an enzyme called alpha-amylase. Because this enzyme is responsible for breaking down amylose starches into simple sugars, fewer simple sugars are released into the blood stream.

Thusly, berries, in general, are an excellent food to have integrated into any diet. Whether dealing with cancer, cardiovascular diseases, such as high blood pressure, Alzheimer's, or cognitive decline, inflammatory conditions like arthritis, or a family history of these disorders, berries would obviously be beneficial. At the same time, their high fiber content positively impacts the digestive system, and supports effective weight management. These facts make berries a clear choice, as an ingredient in a superfood-smoothie.

- Bananas

Bananas are also an important component for smoothies. Not only do they have numerous health benefits, but they add sweetness and creaminess to the texture. Though high in sugar, bananas are included in the low, glycemic index. Their high fiber content, vitamin B6, and biotin properties help the body to regulate blood sugar, making bananas a safe food for people with blood sugar issues. Biotin is also vital for healthy skin, hair, and nails, which explains why it is often added to cosmetic products.

The consumption of biotin, acquired from whole foods, however, provides more of its benefits. As part of the B-complex vitamins (vitamin B7), biotin supports a healthy metabolism, which is critical for achieving optimal weight.

Simultaneously, it is well known that bananas are a major source of potassium, which is an essential mineral for maintaining normal blood pressure and healthy heart function. Since one medium-sized banana contains 400 mg, or more, of potassium, the inclusion of bananas, on a regular basis, can go a long way toward the prevention of high blood pressure and other cardiovascular diseases. Furthermore, bananas are referred to as, "the food of athletes." The reason is that they provide a quick, sustained, and substantial boost of energy to the body. They also contain serotonin, and a chemical called tryptophan, which elevate the mood and fight stress. Consequently, most people report feeling better after eating a banana, as a mid-day snack. It seems to lessen that tired and/or stressed out feeling. The fiber in bananas also facilitates digestion and contributes to the prevention of colon cancer. They are loaded with a variety of nutrients including: vitamin B6 (22% DV), vitamin C (17% DV), folate (6% DV), manganese (16% DV), potassium (12% DV), magnesium (8% DV), copper (10% DV), biotin (10% DV), fiber (12% DV).

- Pineapple

The extraordinary juiciness and intense, tropical flavor of pineapple, which balances the tastes of sweet and tart, make this an excellent fruit, to counter-balance the bitter taste that can come from certain greens, when making power-smoothies. This is one of the secrets for creating delightful green-smoothies.

Pineapples provide a wide range of nutrients, such as B-vitamins, including vitamin B1 (thiamine) (11% DV), B6 (9% DV), B9 (folate) (7% DV), and B5 (pantothenic acid) (7% DV). However, they are exceptionally high in vitamin C (132% DV) and manganese (76% DV). These two nutrients assist the body to stimulate the increase of collagen, which is instrumental in preventing premature aging. Pineapple contains a natural compound, called Bromelain, which provides anti-inflammatory and digestive benefits.

Manganese, on the other hand, aids the body to form connective tissue, and plays a major role in fat and carbohydrate metabolism, calcium absorption, blood sugar regulation, and normal brain and nerve functions. As these elements, all play crucial roles in energy production, the use of pineapple in a superfood-smoothie, is a great way to boost energy.

- Papaya

Papaya is another fruit high in vitamin C (144% DV in 1 cup) and vitamin A (31 % DV). These two nutrients alone provide a wide range of health benefits, such as cardiovascular health, cancer prevention, and immune support. Papaya is a good source of many other nutrients, including the enzymes, papain and chymopapain, which support digestion and reduce inflammation.

- Mangos

High in vitamin C (76% DV) and vitamin A (25% DV), mangos too are excellent sources of vitamin E (9% DV). This percentage of vitamin E is uncommon in most fruits, except avocados. It promotes healthy skin and hormonal levels. Other mango nutrients include: potassium, copper, and B-vitamins. Mangos contain digestive enzymes and other bioactive compounds, which support intestinal health, foster cardiovascular health, cancer prevention (due to the high amount of beta carotene and vitamin C), good vision, healthy skin, and a strong immune system.

- Kiwi

Another source of vitamin C (117% DV) is one peeled, medium kiwi fruit. Kiwi is a good source of fiber (2 g per medium fruit and 9% DV), vitamin K (38% DV), vitamin E (6% DV), folate (5% DV), potassium (7% DV), and copper (5% DV). They are loaded with a wide range of phytonutrients, with the ability to protect DNA in the nucleus of human cells, thus protecting the body from heart diseases, cancers, and premature aging.

The health benefits of kiwi fruit are numerous. A high percentage of vitamin C supports the immune system, protects from infections, such as colds and flu, and aids in relieving respiratory symptoms associated with asthma. Rich in potassium and fiber, eating kiwi supports healthy blood pressure, good digestion, and helps regulate blood sugar levels. Researchers have found that diets rich in fiber also reduce high cholesterol levels, which in turn reduce the risk of heart disease and heart attacks. Additionally, fiber binds and removes toxins from the colon, which is paramount in preventing colon cancer.

Despite all of the kiwi's health benefits, however, not everyone likes it, because of an aftertaste that often comes from eating the seeds. For this reason, adding kiwi to smoothies is a better way to enjoy the health advantages it provides.

- Cherries

Rich in antioxidants, anti-inflammatory compounds, and many other health promoting substances, cherries are a great source of vitamin A (40% DV) and vitamin C (26% DV). They contain significant amounts of potassium (8% DV), copper (8% DV), and manganese (9% DV), and are extremely high in many B-vitamins. There are two primary varieties of cherries: sweet and tart (also known as sour cherries). Tart cherries are often used to make juice concentrates that provide some unique health benefits, including the prevention of obesity and Type 2 diabetes. This is accomplished by activating PPAR (peroxisome proliferator activating receptors) in the body's tissues, which helps to regulate genes involved in fat and glucose metabolism. Additionally, cherries contain natural melatonin, which plays a vital role in sleep. Research suggests that consuming tart, cherry juice not only helps increase melatonin levels, but may improve the quality of one's sleep.

https://www.ncbi.nlm.nih.gov/pmc/articles/PMC3133468/

- **Apricots, Peaches, Nectarines**

Apricots, peaches, and nectarines have many similarities, including their orange color and high levels of beta-carotene, which boosts vision health, the immune system, and protects cells from oxidative damage. These fruits have elevated levels of potassium that promote healthy blood pressure, and vitamin E, which fosters healthy skin, and hormone levels. The high percentage of fiber in these fruits enhances the digestive process and lowers the chances of colon cancer. Apricots, peaches, and nectarines are a good source of B-vitamins and manganese, which are crucial to the body's production of energy. Apricots are a strong dietary source of catechin—a powerful antioxidant and anti-inflammatory compound also found in green tea and linked to cardiovascular health. Lastly, studies have shown that the consumption of foods rich in catechin may help reduce body fat, thus lessening obesity.

https://www.ncbi.nlm.nih.gov/pubmed/15640470

- Avocados

Avocados are a powerhouse of vitamins, minerals, and phytonutrients. They are extremely high in mono-unsaturated fat ("good" fat), as well as a notable source of omega-3 fatty acid—all linked to cardiovascular health. Avocados contain such nutrients as: potassium, vitamin K, vitamin C, vitamin E, fiber, phosphorus, copper, magnesium, manganese, zinc, and all B vitamins, except B12. The addition of avocados to an already well-balanced diet has been shown to lower the risk of heart disease, improve blood levels with LDL cholesterol, and lessen oxidative stress in the bloodstream. They support satiety, control blood sugar and insulin regulation, all of which are good for weight management. Added to smoothies, avocados not only boost the nutrition profile, but provide a smooth texture to the drink.

Although these are the fruits I tend to incorporate most in my smoothies, it does not exclude the use of other fruits, such as apples, pears, grapes, cantaloupe, honey dew, and/or watermelon. Any fruit can be used to make superfood-smoothies. It would be advisable, however, to use fruits, or vegetables, that you are less likely to eat on their own. In that way, you will expand the variety of foods in your diet. This is key to improving the nutrient intake for your body's optimal health.

Chapter Nine
Superfood Smoothies 101

❖❖❖❖❖❖

F or any process to attain maximum success, it is important to use the best products and tools or equipment. When making superfood smoothies that are well mixed and blended, the following equipment is recommended:

- Blender

Any common, everyday blender, with a minimum 600-watt motor, can do the job. If cost is an issue, a blender of this type will ultimately enable you to create a delicious drink, as directed, but it will take a little longer, because it is necessary to blend your smoothie in stages, especially when using frozen fruits. This is so the machine will work efficiently and not burn out the motor. I have had good success with Oster brands: the Oster 600-Watt Fusion Blender (model BRLY07-B00-000) (about $60), and the

Oster Reverse Crush Counterforms Blender (about $40) have worked effectively. Furthermore, the Hamilton Beach's Wave Crusher Multi-Function Blender, with 14 Speeds, has proved to be good choice that only costs about $30.

Nevertheless, you will achieve the best results with a heavy-duty blender (emulsifier), such as Vitamix, Ninja Professional Blender, Blendtec, or NutriBullet. The size of the NutriBullet is an especially convenient alternative for people who travel. Although, these are more expensive choices, a heavy-duty machine of this type has the power to make a truly smooth drink, in a fraction of the time. Its power allows you to add all the ingredients at the same time, cutting down on prep time.

Either way, when choosing your appliance, look for one with a heavy base, a large pitcher—at least 40 ounces—and the most blending power you can afford. The heavy base prevents shaking, when blending frozen fruits, and a large pitcher allows you to make a bigger batch that can be saved for later use.

- Citrus Press

A citrus press, or lemon squeezer, is inexpensive and easy to use, although electric citrus juicers are also commercially available.

- ## Chopping Board

Always keep a separate cutting board for preparing fruits and vegetables. Never use it for poultry, meat, or fish.

- ## Knife

Select a knife that you are comfortable using for peeling fruits and chopping vegetables.

- ## 16 or 32-oz Glass Jars with Air-tight Lids

Mason jars work particularly well for storing smoothies for later use.

- ## Baking Sheets

Baking sheets can be used to freeze fruits, before transferring them into freezer bags. That will be mentioned more in the "tips" section.

- ## Parchment Paper

Parchment paper is the best thing to use for covering the baking sheets, before arranging cut fruit to store in the freezer.

These are the basic items needed to start making your superfood-smoothies. As you progress, you may identify ideas that require other equipment.

How to Make a Superfood-Smoothie

When you first start making smoothies, you may be tempted to use more fruit that make it overly sweet. However, you should keep in mind that too much sugar from fruit can raise your blood sugar, which can be a problem for people with diabetes, or insulin resistance.

After trying many different combinations, I have found one basic formula that has worked for all my clients, including those with diabetes. I realize that, particularly in the beginning, to enjoy your smoothie, it must be somewhat sweet. My formula, therefore, produces a smoothie that is sweet enough for most people. You must keep in mind, however, that enjoying superfood-smoothies is an acquired taste—the more you drink them, the more you will like them. Ultimately, you will even crave them, and you will notice a decrease in sugar cravings, because your taste buds will become increasingly accustomed to more moderate sweetness.

The following basic formula makes about 40-60 ounces of smoothie that you can divide into two or three daily servings:

- 2 cups green leafy vegetables, or two big handfuls
- 2 cups liquid or more if needed
- Some 'good' fat, from nuts, seeds, nut butter, or avocado
- 1½ cups mixed fruits

- ½ cup frozen bananas, or one medium banana, if using fresh
- Some protein, such as whey, plant protein...(optional).
- Any other superfoods (optional)

Depending on the fruits used in the recipe, I do not always add extra sweeteners to my smoothies. Sweetness from fruit varies, and sometimes added protein tends to cut down on the sweetness provided by fruits. In that case, if a little more sweetness is desired, add one to two tablespoons of raw honey, blackstrap molasses, or one to three soft dates, such as Medjool dates—pitted and chopped. The addition of a little more banana is also an option, if you don't mind that taste being noticeable. Personally, I don't want all my smoothies to taste like banana. I, therefore, discovered that using a half cup of banana or one medium banana provides the desired sweetness and creaminess, without much detectible banana flavor. It is also OK to replace that half cup of banana with another sweet fruit of your choosing.

Liquids for your Smoothies

Water is the basic liquid to be used in making a smoothie, and it does not add any extra calories. However, milk does enhance the taste of a smoothie and boosts the nutritional profile. Dairy milk is one of the most nourishing foods on the earth, since it contains almost all the nutrients needed by the human body. It is a great source of protein, with 8 grams in just one cup. Milk is also high in calcium, potassium, phosphorus. Nevertheless, for some reason, there are people who cannot digest milk properly, or have other medical conditions that can be aggravated by milk. In that case, non-dairy milk such as almond milk is a good alternative.

Besides Water and Milk, or Milk Substitutes, other liquids can be used in smoothies that include:

- Coconut water
- Freshly squeezed orange juice
- Cranberry juice
- Pomegranate juice
- cherry juice
- Brewed tea

Coconut water is a delightful, hydrating drink packed with nutrients. It is especially high in naturally occurring electrolytes, such as potassium, magnesium, sodium, phosphorus, and calcium. It is no wonder that some marketers refer to it as "nature's sports drink." Electrolytes are nutrients present in the body that have important functions, such as maintaining water balance and normal PH, and regulating the heartbeat, blood pressure, and electrical signals in the brain and muscles.

Consequently, if high blood pressure is an issue, coconut water is a good choice. One cup of coconut water actually contains more potassium than a banana. It also brings a tropical, sweet kick to a smoothie that is very refreshing.

When choosing coconut water, or any of the juices listed above, be certain to check the ingredient list for added sugars. Simply using any type of fruit juice in a smoothie is not always the best idea. Alternatively, cranberry, pomegranate, and cherry juices are often recommended, because the whole fruits are not always in season. Using pure 100% juice, from these fruits, is a good way to enjoy their numerous health benefits, when available.

Freshly squeezed orange juice is primarily encouraged, for orange based recipes. Furthermore, many teas are often loaded with antioxidants and can provide other health benefits as well. For that reason, do not hesitate to add tea to your diet. You can brew a cup, or two, to drink, and then use the remainder as part of the liquid in a smoothie.

NOTES

Chapter Ten
Protein in Your Smoothie

❖❖❖❖❖❖

*P*roteins are the building blocks that the body uses to maintain healthy structure and growth of body tissue—including development and repair. Hair, skin, eyes, muscles, and organs are all made from protein. They are critical for numerous biochemical processes in the body; and amino acids are their building blocks.

Although there are 20 amino acids that the body can't live without, it only manufactures 11 of them. The rest of those needed must be gotten from one's diet. This type of amino acid is known as 'essential amino acids'. In addition to the growth functions mentioned, protein is also a source of energy, along with carbohydrates and fat. In general, animal proteins like meat, dairy, and eggs contain all essential amino acids, but most plant foods contain different combinations of them.

Considering how critical protein is to the body, you might be wondering how much is needed, on a daily basis. This depends upon several factors—age, sex, muscle mass, activity levels, and current state of health. The DRI (Dietary Reference Intake) is 0.8 grams of protein per kilogram of body weight, or 0.36 grams per pound. If you are just trying to stay healthy, simply eating quality proteins in your meals, along with other nutritious foods, should bring your intake to that optimal range.

Why add extra protein to smoothies?

While it is true that greens and other ingredients in smoothies provide protein, it is not enough to satisfy the recommended daily requirements for a complete meal. If you are using a smoothie as a meal replacement, it will be necessary to boost the protein content, by adding some additional protein supplement, or another high protein food to reach a recommended level. Protein is imperative to the growth of muscle, as well as controlling the appetite, keeping you satiated, and preventing blood sugar spikes. Consuming a smoothie, without added protein, will not adequately satisfy that need. While you may feel full immediately upon consuming it, before long you start feeling hungry again. Also, if you have diabetes, are insulin resistant, or are trying to lose weight and/or maintain a healthy weight, adding extra protein to a smoothie is highly recommended. Furthermore, when exercising regularly, adding protein to the smoothie will support the growth of lean muscle mass.

Protein Options:

- **Whey Protein Powder**

Whey protein is very popular among athletes and bodybuilders, because it is great for promoting muscle growth and maintenance, when coupled with strength training. However, besides protein, whey also contains a combination of beneficial bioactive compounds that aid in lowering blood pressure levels and promoting vascular relaxation, without the side effects of drugs. The consumption, particularly of grass-fed protein, supports healthy lipid levels and immune system response.

Whey protein is one of the two proteins found in milk, with the other being casein. During cheese production, a coagulant (usually the enzyme rennet) is added to milk, and the liquid whey is separated from the curds (casein). Whey protein is a complete, high-quality protein, very digestible, and absorbs into the system quickly, as compared to many other types of protein. Additionally, it contains essential amino acids. These qualities make whey one of the best protein supplements available. The two common types of whey protein are: whey protein concentrate and whey protein isolate.

Whey protein concentrate typically contains about 60–80% protein, with the remaining 20–30% from fat and carbs. Whey protein isolates go through another process that removes fat and carbs—further concentrating the protein. Protein isolate powders contain about 90–95% protein. If you happen to be lactose intolerant, whey protein isolate is more suitable than concentrate, since this extra processing removes most of the lactose. When choosing a protein powder, make certain it is from grass-fed cows that are not fed hormones or antibiotics. This assures a better quality than protein from conventionally raised cows.

- **Collagen Hydrolysate AKA Collagen Peptides**

Collagen is the most abundant type of protein found in the human body. The basic texture of this element is known as gelatin, and is made by cooking the bones, connective tissues, skin, and tendons of animals. The resulting product is called collagen, and has many uses. In the food industry, it is that derivative used to make deserts, such as 'jello' and puddings, because they gel when mixed with hot liquid, and then set-up jiggly (like jello), when chilled.

Like all proteins, collagen is comprised of amino acids—glycine and proline being the primary ones. To make gelatin powder, the collagen is dried and further processed, using enzymes to break the bonds between the amino acids, thus leaving the amino acids intact. This processed, end-product is known as collagen hydrolysate, or collagen peptides. Because the amino acids are further broken down, some people find collagen hydrolysate easier to digest. Collagen hydrolysate doesn't thicken when added to hot or cold liquid, making it convenient to add to your smoothies. Health wise, collagen is the compound responsible for giving skin elasticity, hair its strength, and connective tissue its ability to hold everything in place. It is like the glue that keeps our parts held together.

Unfortunately, collagen degrades with age, as do many elements of the body, leaving us vulnerable to achy joints, sore muscles, and wrinkled skin. Collagen facilitates joint mobility, reduces arthritic pain, helps heal leaky gut syndrome, and relieve the discomfort associated with IBS and other gastrointestinal disorders. It also boosts metabolism and muscle mass, increases energy, and supports cardiovascular health, by strengthening blood vessels and improving their elasticity. Collagen improves liver function, due to the presence of glycine, an amino acid that minimizes damage to the liver experienced by the absorption of toxins or alcohol. Collagen also supports healthy blood sugar; and has been shown to prevent wrinkles, promote healthy hair and nails, and stimulate the healing of wounds. So go ahead and add some collagen hydrolysate to your smoothies, to boost your health and beauty.

Most collagen supplements on the market are from conventionally raised beef, treated with antibiotics and hormones. It is important to look for collagen sourced from grass-fed cows, to ensure the highest quality. Be certain the ingredient list also reflects no additives or unwanted fillers.

- ### Egg Protein Powder

Egg protein powder is not as popular as whey. Nevertheless, it is a beneficial protein supplement. Made from egg whites, egg protein is a complete protein; therefore, providing adequate amounts of the nine essential amino acids the body does not produce. It is lactose-free, so it too is a good substitute for anyone who is lactose intolerant.

- ### Soy Protein Powder

Soy protein powder is one of the rare plant proteins considered as a 'complete protein', because it contains the essential amino acids that the body requires. This is the reason why soy products are particularly popular among vegetarians. Soy protein further contains other nutrients and phytochemicals, such as isoflavones, which are proven to promote cardiovascular health and aid in cancer prevention. When buying soy products, it is good to choose organic, considering that 94% of soy crops grown in the United States are genetically modified—according to the US Department of Agriculture.

https://www.ers.usda.gov/data-products/adoption-of-genetically-engineered-crops-in-the-us/recent-trends-in-ge-adoption.aspx

- Green Soybeans

Also known as 'edamame', green soybeans are the fresh soybeans, which are often found in the frozen vegetable sections of grocery stores. One cup of green soybeans contains 17 grams of complete protein, which is an incredibly high amount coming from a plant food. They also provide a wide range of other nutrients, including 8 grams of fiber, 79% DV of manganese, 25% DV of magnesium, 20% DV of iron, 19% DV of potassium, 26% DV of phosphorus, 10% DV of calcium, 52% DV of vitamin K, 16% DV of vitamin C, 21% DV of thiamine, 14% DV of riboflavin, 7% DV of niacin, 8% DV of B6, and 21% DV of folate. All these nutrients come with only 189 calories. Edamame, too, contains high levels and a variety, of phytonutrients, including isoflavones, phytoestrogen (plant estrogen), and polyphenols.

There are many health benefits in this food, including the reduction of menopause symptoms and prevention of calcium loss, which is linked to osteoporosis. Research has shown that isoflavones likewise help reduce both overall cholesterol levels and LDL cholesterol, or "bad" cholesterol.

https://www.ncbi.nlm.nih.gov/pubmed/24473985

- Tofu

Made from soy milk, Tofu is called the 'cheese of Asia', because the methods used to produce it are like those used to make cheese. Tofu is high in protein, with 8 grams in each 3.5-oz (100-gram) serving. Since tofu is made from soy milk, it offers all of the nutrients and health benefits of soybeans mentioned above. Tofu is tasteless by itself, and often takes on the flavor of other ingredients, when combined in a recipe. Therefore, it blends well in a smoothie and gives a creamy texture to the drink. If you are not allergic to soy products, and you can get past the controversies surrounding soy, tofu is a good alternative source of protein to add to a smoothie recipe.

- Pea Protein Powder

Pea protein powder is relatively new, but especially popular among vegetarians and people with allergies, or sensitivities, to dairy, soy, or egg products. It is made from the yellow split pea and is a high-fiber legume that contains all the essential amino acids the body requires. Though many people have problems digesting legumes, pea protein powder is highly digestible, and does not give the discomfort often associated with split peas, or other legumes.

- Hemp Protein Powder

Hemp protein is not only a good source of protein—easily digested by the body—it is also a good source of nutrients, such as fiber, omega-3 fatty acid, Vitamin E, calcium, iron, cooper, magnesium, potassium, and phosphorus. It is a complete protein, containing all nine essential amino acids. The nutritional profile of this protein makes it a great supplement that bolsters the immune system, promotes heart health, and balances blood sugar.

- Brown Rice Protein Powder

Alone, brown rice does not provide all nine essential amino acids. Therefore, brown rice protein powder is often blended with another protein, such as quinoa or chia, to form a complete protein. Nevertheless, the nutrition profile of brown rice protein is not limited to protein. It also provides 'good' fat, fiber, iron, calcium, and antioxidants.

- ## Mixed Plant Protein

As we mentioned earlier, most plant proteins are also low in one or more amino acids needed by the body. However, choosing a blend of plant types is very beneficial. There are some companies that even add nuts and seeds to their protein blends, which provides more nutrients than in plant mixes alone

- ## Plain Greek Yogurt

Greek yogurt is a very thick type of yogurt made by straining regular yogurt to remove the whey, or watery part. Because this straining process removes some carbohydrates, Greek yogurt is thicker and higher in protein. It is typically lower in both sugar and carbohydrates than standard yogurts, and non-fat, or low-fat, varieties contain the most protein with fewer calories. It is, therefore, a better choice to boost the protein content in smoothies.

Along with enhancing the protein content of a smoothie, Greek yogurt gives it a creamy texture and contains the nutrients found in milk. As a further benefit, it provides useful bacteria to the body, and functions as a probiotic, supporting intestinal health. This too boosts the immune system. When selecting a yogurt, however, it is important to look for the words "live and active cultures," which indicate that the yogurt has living bacteria. When buying yogurt, it is best to choose organic whenever possible. This avoids exposure to growth hormones and antibiotics contained in some yogurts made from conventional milk.

- Cottage Cheese

Cottage cheese is soft and creamy with a mild flavor. It is considered a fresh cheese, so it does not undergo an aging process to develop its flavor. Often recommended as part of a healthy diet, its popularity has grown in the past few decades. Available in creamed, whipped, lactose-free, reduced sodium, and reduced fat varieties, cottage cheese is a powerhouse of protein. One cup (226 grams) of cottage cheese, with 2% fat, contains 27 grams of protein and is high in calcium, phosphorus, potassium, selenium, Vitamin B2 (Riboflavin), and B12—with only 194 calories. Cottage cheese is a good addition to smoothie for both its creamy texture and high nutrient profile. It is recommended to select a low sodium and low-fat variety, if possible, as well as organic.

- ## Nut Butter and Powder

A very popular protein is nut butter, and of the various types, peanut butter is favorite. Not only does it taste good, but it is loaded with many nutrients, including protein. Two tablespoons of peanut butter contain 7-8 grams of protein and 200 calories. Peanut powder, however, is a great alternative, because it tastes just like peanut butter, but has a lower fat and calorie content. Two tablespoons of peanut powder have 5-6 grams of protein with only 45-50 calories. This is particularly important, if you are trying to reduce calorie intake and lose weight. Almond butter is another suitable source of protein, with 6 grams of protein in two tablespoons, and 167-210 calories. Besides containing protein, these nut butters and powders are good sources of antioxidants, fiber, good fat, vitamins, and minerals.

- ## Beans and peas

All legumes (beans, lentils, soybeans, and peas) are excellent sources of protein, fiber, antioxidants, and many other nutrients, including B vitamins, iron, zinc, magnesium, and potassium. The high protein and fiber content of legumes make them important to regulating blood sugar, reducing LDL cholesterol, and supporting weight loss. Their whole nutritional profile provides many additional health benefits, such as cancer prevention and cardiovascular support. Legumes are particularly recommended for use in smoothies. Sweet peas are a good place to start, since they pair well with the sweetness of fruit.

- Oats

Finally, oats are among the healthiest grains available. They are high in protein and loaded with antioxidants, fibers, vitamins, and minerals. They contain large quantities of beta-glucan, a type of soluble fiber that forms a gel-like substance in the gut. Though beta-glucan fiber has been found to reduce LDL and total cholesterol levels, regulate blood sugar and insulin production, increase satiety, which is important for weight loss, and promote growth of good bacteria in the digestive tract, it also seems to heighten the immune system. One-half cup of Old-fashioned, rolled oats has 7 grams of protein, 5 grams of fiber, and 190 calories. When choosing oats for smoothies, it is good to know that rolled oats have a creamier texture than steel-cut oats, and are most recommended.

Conclusion

As you experiment with protein sources that sound good, or you already enjoy, try them in your smoothie recipes. It will help you to determine which you like and serve you best. Remember, however, to rotate the types of protein used, since the body benefits from variety.

Chapter Eleven
Super-Charge Your Smoothie with Superfoods

❖❖❖❖❖❖

*T*he term 'superfood' has become a popular catchword in the health food industry; it is often used to describe any food that is incredibly high in nutrients and/or known to help with specific health issues. The consumption of these foods has been proven to lower risk of cancer and heart disease, as well as promote overall health and vitality. Some of them even provide relief for specific symptoms. These are the types of superfoods we like to add to our smoothies.

For instance, when it comes to arthritis pain, turmeric has been shown to be as effective in relieving the symptoms, as the anti-inflammatory drug, Ibuprofen. Another example of superfood is Acerola cherry—an exotic fruit incredibly high in vitamin C. When talking about Vitamin C, what usually comes to mind are oranges. However, one teaspoon of acerola cherry provides almost twenty times the vitamin C, of an orange, with only 10 calories. A medium orange provides 93% of DV of vitamin C, with 62 calories. Therefore, to get the same amount of vitamin C from oranges, you would need to consume at least 19 oranges, with 1,178 calories. Thusly, to increase your vitamin C intake, acerola cherry is a better choice than oranges. Adding these superfoods to a smoothie, in powdered form, allows you to enjoy the health benefits of some very beneficial foods that you might otherwise not consume.

Let's take a quick look at some of my favorite superfoods:

- ### Nuts and Seeds

Nuts and seeds—almonds, Brazil nuts, pecans, cashews, walnuts, and pistachios, and seeds—pumpkin, sunflower, and sesame seeds, are nutrient powerhouses. Added to a smoothie, in their raw form, provides even greater benefits. Packed with protein, heart supporting fats and fiber, most nuts and seeds are also particularly high in minerals—magnesium, manganese, phosphorus, cooper, zinc, and selenium, as well as vitamins and antioxidants. The synergistic effects of these nutrients stabilize blood sugar, lower total and LDL cholesterol, plus triglycerides, while boosting levels of HDL cholesterol. They help to balance hormones, boost the immune system, promote energy production, support healthy skin, and decrease cravings for unhealthy foods.

Although all nuts and seeds provide similar nutrients and health benefits, each has its own unique quality. For instance, the Brazil nut is extremely high in selenium—only 2-3 Brazil nuts provide 100% DV. Pumpkin seeds are one of the richest, natural sources of tryptophan, which, when converted by the body into serotonin and then melatonin, is known as 'the sleep hormone.' Pumpkin seeds have long been valued as a source of the mineral zinc, which the World Health Organization recommends as a good way to obtain this nutrient. Compared to other nuts, walnuts are higher in omega-3 fatty acid; sunflower seeds have high contents of vitamin E, B-complex vitamins, and many other minerals (1/4 cup provides 82% of vitamin E, 70% of copper, and 43% vitamin B3); and sesame seeds are an incredibly important source of copper—163% DV in ¼ cup.

- **Flaxseed, Chia Seed, Hemp Seed**

What flaxseed, chia seed, and hemp seed have in common is their extremely high content of omega-3 fatty acid, when compared to other foods. However, flaxseed surpasses them, by being the number one source of alpha-linolenic acid (ALA), a plant-based omega-3 fatty acid. These fatty acids are known for their anti-inflammatory properties, and, as we mentioned in previous chapters, chronic inflammation has been linked to most degenerative diseases. Therefore, including these seeds in your diet can be very beneficial. Alpha-linolenic acid converts into small amounts of an EPA and DHA form of Omega-3's—the ones found in fish that are crucial to a healthy heart and good brain functions.

Besides being high in Omega-3 fatty acids, each of these seeds has its own particularity, even though flaxseed and chia seeds have some similarities. They are both high in a type of water-soluble fiber called "mucilage". This gel-forming fiber prevents blood sugar spikes, by preventing stomach contents from emptying too rapidly into the small intestine. Mucilage fiber also helps to lower LDL cholesterol, which is known as "bad cholesterol." This is possible without the drug side effects of statins and other "cholesterol lowering" medications.

Flaxseed, however, has something that hemp and chia seeds don't have; it contains lignans, phytochemicals, which have been linked to the prevention of breast and prostate cancer. Some studies suggest that lignans in flaxseed may also reduce hot flashes associated with menopause. To gain the nutritional benefits of flax, the seeds must be ground; otherwise, whole flaxseeds pass through your intestinal tract undigested. Ground flaxseed should be kept in an airtight jar in the refrigerator, to prevent the oil from becoming rancid. Hemp and chia seeds can be eaten whole or ground.

Hemp seed, on the other hand, outshines chia and flaxseed, when it comes to protein, with 10g per three tablespoons (one serving size). Moreover, the protein in hemp seeds contains all of the essential amino acids, which is uncommon in plant foods. As mentioned previously, amino acids are the building blocks of protein, and essential amino acids must be in your diet, because the body cannot manufacture all of them on its own. Additionally, these seeds are an excellent source of elements, such as calcium, magnesium, iron, zinc, phosphorous, and manganese. Bottom line, the body benefits from having any of these three seeds, as a part of a diet. To maximize their benefits, it is important to rotate them, since each has something unique to offer.

- Black Seeds

Black seeds (Nigella sativa) are believed to be indigenous to the Mediterranean region, but have been cultivated in other parts of the world, including Northern Africa and Asia. It is referred to as black cumin, black caraway, black sesame, onion seed, and Roman coriander. In Arabic cultures, black seed is known as "Habbatul barakah", meaning the "seed of blessing." It is also believed that the Islamic prophet, Mohammed, said it was "a cure for all diseases except death." This claim made black seeds popular among Muslims, as a remedy for many health ailments, including asthma, bronchitis, allergies, and other respiratory conditions.

The popularity of black seeds, as a 'cure-all', has raised interest among scientists over the years. Hundreds of peer-reviewed articles have been published that confirm many of the claims made about these 'miraculous' seeds. Scientists have found more than 100 chemical compounds in black seeds that work collectively to regulate the immune system. This might then explain the power of black seed on so many health ailments. Recent research has provided evidence that most illnesses arise due to an imbalanced, or dysfunctional, immune system, which cannot perform its primary functions. Back seed is therefore very helpful when dealing with auto-immune disorders, including rheumatoid arthritis.

Studies have also shown powerful anti-tumor and anti-microbial activities in black seeds, including multidrug-resistant bacteria.

These powerful seeds also support the liver's health, by preventing both damage and disease. Black seeds may also have an impact on digestive disorders, skin diseases, urinary and reproductive system infections. They may help balance blood sugar levels, regulate cholesterol and blood pressure.

Adding black seeds to a smoothie is a convenient way to enjoy these health benefits. Black seed oil can, also, be used in a smoothie, in place of the whole seeds—both offer similar health benefits.

- Turmeric

Turmeric has been used in India for thousands of years, as a spice and medicinal herb. Now that science has proven many of the health benefits that the Indians have known for ages, turmeric has also become popular in the western world. Countless, peer-reviewed articles substantiate these findings. Curcumin is the primary ingredient in turmeric, and has powerful, anti-inflammatory effects, as well as being a strong antioxidant.

In numerous studies, turmeric has been compared to some very common medications used to treat specific conditions, with impressive results. For instance, the anti-inflammatory effects of turmeric have been shown to be comparable to the over-the-counter, anti-inflammatory agent, Motrin. Turmeric's combination of antioxidant and anti-inflammatory effects explains why many people experience relief from the pain of arthritis, when the spice is used on a regular basis.

I have personally experienced the anti-inflammatory effect of turmeric with my daughter. She had all her wisdom teeth removed on a Friday, and on Monday, she was back to school completely pain free. Her classmates couldn't believe it.

While several friends had had the same procedure before, their experience had been completely different. She came home from the dentist with two different pain medications and an ice pack, but she never used any of it. Her recovering process was faster than anticipated, even by the doctor. All I gave her was an "anti-inflammatory juice" (recipe included in this book), and every time I checked to see if she needed the pain medication, the answer was "No." The night of her procedure, she was able to eat solid food, with no pain or inflammation. The only thing we used from the doctor was the mouth rinse solution. That is the power of turmeric. My daughter has also successfully used turmeric, along with ginger, to control menstrual pain. This has replaced her usual dose of Ibuprofen.

Turmeric also provides support for brain health, by increasing the growth of new neurons, fights various degenerative processes in the brain, supports cardiovascular health and the immune system, aids in lowering blood cholesterol, and improves the balance of blood sugars. In addition, turmeric is well known as antimicrobial, antibacterial, antifungal, antiviral, analgesic, and may prevent and support the treatment of many types of cancer. Turmeric is one of those things you want to have in your diet, and adding it to a smoothie makes that easy!

- ## Unsulphured Blackstrap Molasses

Blackstrap molasses is a thick, syrup by-product, of the process of refining sugar cane into table sugar. It is obtained, after the third boiling of the syrup remaining, when the sugar's sucrose has been crystallized. It is, therefore, more concentrated than other molasses. Although used as a sweetener, blackstrap molasses contains less sugar than table sugar, and the taste is somewhat bittersweet. Unlike refined white sugar and corn syrup, which provide empty calories, blackstrap molasses is a healthful sweetener that contains impressive amounts of a variety of minerals. It is particularly concentrated in iron, potassium, manganese, magnesium, copper, calcium, selenium and zinc, and is rich in vitamin B6 and antioxidants.

Blackstrap molasses has been used to overcome anemia, because of its high iron concentration, which is essential for creating red blood cells. It may also address issues of high blood pressure, high LDL, chronic fatigue, ADHD, and depression. Surprisingly, this sugary substance may act to stabilize blood sugar, in people with diabetes or insulin resistance.

Adding blackstrap molasses to your diet should be a major consideration. Its nutrients are in their natural, balanced form, creating a nutritional synergy that synthetic supplements cannot equal. It you are trying to boost your iron intake, I highly recommend adding blackstrap molasses to your smoothie. A benefit of making your own smoothies is that you can select nutrient-dense foods that meet your specific needs, and mix them together into a drink that you enjoy. Adding blackstrap molasses to your drinks not only boosts the nutrition profile of your smoothies, but adds a touch of sweetness.

- Moringa leaves powder

Moringa leaves are another of nature's highly nutritious foods. The plant is often referred to as the 'Miracle Tree', for all parts are usable— either for food or medicine. It is rare for a single plant to contain many essential nutrients and furthermore in high quantities. However, research has shown that the moringa has a higher content of different nutrients compared to those found individually in several different types of food and vegetables. For instance 100 grams of moringa leaves contain:

- 10 times the vitamin A of carrots
- 12 times the vitamin C of oranges
- 17 times the calcium of milk
- 15 times the potassium of bananas
- 9 times the protein of yogurt

Moringa is also a rich source of complete protein, having all nine essential amino acids. Due to its high nutrition profile, and the ease of growing it—even in poor soil—moringa is often promoted in some underprivileged countries, to fight hunger and prevent malnutrition.

Throughout the world, moringa is used to address a variety of conditions, including diabetes, chronic fatigue, anemia, fluid retention, thyroid disorders, digestive problems and inflammation-related diseases, such as arthritis. Today studies have confirmed these health benefits of moringa.

Its high percentage of antioxidants and anti-inflammatory phytonutrients give moringa cancer and heart disease prevention properties. In powder form, moringa leaf is a whole food, meaning its abundant nutrients are more efficiently absorbed and utilized by the body. This is unlike many conventional supplements and multi-vitamins. So go ahead and create your own natural supplement by adding moringa leaves powder to your smoothies.

- Matcha Green Tea

Matcha Powder is a unique type of tea made from whole, Japanese green tea leaves that is renowned for its multiple health benefits. During the last few weeks before harvest, green tea leaves are shaded from the sun, increasing their chlorophyll content and creating a beautiful green color. Upon picking, the leaves are carefully ground with stone grinding wheels, to produce a fine powder. The process, of grinding the whole leaves into a super fine powder, yields a higher concentration of nutrients.

Matcha green tea is great source of antioxidant, and is exceptionally high in catechins, a type of polyphenol, also abundant in flaxseed, as well as chlorophyll, often abundant in most green plants. The concentration of catechins in matcha powder, however, has been shown to increase the rate of utilization of stored fat, as energy. It, furthermore, decreases the formation of new fat cells. Additionally, matcha significantly effects the lowering of LDL cholesterol, thus protecting the body from heart disease. The high concentration of chlorophyll supports detoxification, and protects cells from oxidative damages linked to cancer, rapid aging, and other degenerative diseases. Finally, matcha contains L-theanine, an amino acid known to relax the mind. For this reason, matcha is viewed as a mood enhancer.

- ## Wheat Grass

In the past few years, wheat grass (*triticum aestivum)* has become popular among health food enthusiasts. If you are on a gluten-free diet, you may wonder if there is any gluten in wheat grass. The answer is "No!" Wheat grass is a gluten-free food.

Wheat grass is a popular add-in, at smoothie and juice bars, because it provides concentrated amounts of vitamins, minerals, amino acids, and phytonutrients. It is also a rich source of chlorophyll—a substance that allows plants to absorb energy from sunlight. Chlorophyll has a similar chemical composition to that of hemoglobin. It, therefore, strengthens the blood and provides a boost in energy. Chlorophyll is a natural, liver cleanser and detoxifier, a powerful antioxidant that reduces free radical damage, and assists in the prevention of cancer, heart disease, and other chronic conditions. Because wheat grass is not something generally found in grocery stores, most people, who consume it, either grow it themselves, or use the powder form in their smoothies. Wheat grass powder is available at most health food stores.

- Barley Grass

Just like wheat grass, barley grass is a powerhouse of vitamins, minerals, amino acids, and antioxidants, including beta carotene and chlorophyll. The amazing nutritional profile of barley grass makes it an important food for detoxifying the body, boosting energy, and supporting the immune system. Including barley grass in your diet can improve overall health and reduce the early onset of degenerative diseases. Nevertheless, like wheat grass, barley grass is not easily found in grocery stores. Thusly, you will either need to grow it yourself, or look for a powdered form at a health food store.

- Acai Berry

The acai berry is one of the top nutrient-dense superfoods in the world. Native to South America, acai is a fruit high in anthocyanins, which are a type of flavonoid, with antioxidant effects. Found naturally in many fruits and vegetables, anthocyanins are the pigments that give red, purple, and blue plants their rich coloring. Like such fruits as blueberries, blackberries, Concord grapes, and raspberries, acai have one of the highest ratings, on the ORAC scale (Oxygen Radical Absorbance Capacity). The ORAC scale is a test that measures the antioxidant levels in food. Among these fruits, known for their high antioxidant content, however, there is a huge difference in the ORAC score—e.g. 9,621 for blueberries and 102,700 for acai berries.

This high concentration of anthocyanins, have been shown to support memory and cognitive functions, due to their fatty acid content. They also support the cardiovascular system, as well as prevent premature aging and many degenerative diseases. The "French Paradox"—a French theory about the unexplainable inconsistency between the rate of heart disease, as opposed to the level of consumption of saturated fats in the French diet—attributes anthocyanin, called resveratrol and found in red wine, to be what protects the French from heart disease. Acai has 30 times more anthocyanins than red wine. So, you can enjoy those same benefits derived from red wine, without having to drink it.

- Goji Berry

Goji berry, also known as "wolfberry fruit," is a relative of the tomato, and a natural source of lycopene—a powerful phytonutrient that contributes to the prevention of prostate cancer. For thousands of years, goji berries (Lycium Barbarum) have been revered for their astounding array of potential health benefits. They have been traditionally used as a wholesome food to aid in the overall strengthening of the body. Like the benefits of eating other berries, goji berries are loaded with antioxidants that protect the cells from damage caused by free radicals. Additionally, goji berries support cardiovascular health, brain function, and the immune system. They may also help regulate blood glucose and cholesterol levels, as well as guard against premature aging.

- Ginger

Like turmeric, ginger is an extremely healthful spice that has been used for medicinal purposes, in many cultures around the world. It is loaded with nutrients and bioactive compounds that have powerful benefits on most organs of the body, including the heart and brain. The unique fragrance and flavor of ginger come from its natural oils—the most important of which is gingerol. It is also responsible for many of its medicinal properties.

It has anti-inflammatory and antioxidant effects. Ginger root, long known as a digestive aid, helps relieve many digestive conditions, including the nausea and vomiting often experienced by patients undergoing chemotherapy. It has been proven to be as effective at relieving headaches, arthritis pain, and menstrual cramps, as the common over-the-counter drug, Ibuprofen. Additionally, ginger root may help regulate blood sugar and cholesterol levels. This is also a powerful expectorant that promotes drainage of mucus from the lungs, by thinning the mucus, and lubricating an irritated respiratory tract. It supports cardiovascular health, by relaxing smooth muscle cells, for proper circulation and healthy blood pressure. In smoothies, I usually combine turmeric and ginger, not only for a synergetic benefit, but also for taste.

- Cinnamon

Cinnamon is another spice that has been used medicinally for thousands of years. It is packed with a variety of protective antioxidants that reduce free radical damage and slow the aging process. Among many other health benefits, cinnamon is most known for its blood sugar support, by facilitating the body's use of insulin, as well as the prevention of Type 2 diabetes. Like berries, cacao powder, and red wine, cinnamon contains polyphenols phytonutrients that promote cardiovascular and brain health. These compounds stabilize blood pressure, provide anti-cancer benefits, reduce levels of total cholesterol, LDL, and triglycerides, while HDL, 'good cholesterol' remains stable.

- Raw Cacao Powder

Chocolate is known worldwide, as a delightful, mood-lifting treat. It is made from the cacao bean, and is shown to be a highly, healthful food. However, the processing at high temperatures, as well as the addition of sugar, diminishes some of the benefits of this superfood. Raw cacao powder, on the other hand, is minimally processed and contains many phytochemicals, especially polyphenol antioxidants, which are highly acclaimed for their cardiovascular, health benefits. In comparison by weight, cacao has more antioxidant polyphenols than blueberries, red wine, or black and green teas. Cacao powder is also a very good source of minerals, for example magnesium, manganese, calcium, potassium, selenium, phosphorus, cooper, and zinc.

Studies suggest that the nutrients in cacao powder, along with the variety of phytonutrients, synergistically provide health benefits, such as lowering cholesterol, regulating blood pressure, improving vascular function, and glucose metabolism. What most appeals to people, besides taste, is the positive effect on emotions and mood that raw cacao powder has, by elevating serotonin levels. It contains a neurotransmitter called theobromine—a mild stimulant sometimes used as a treatment for depression. This superfood stimulates the secretion of endorphins, which induce pleasurable feelings—explaining why we often turn to chocolate when feeling distressed. Cacao powder is easy to add to your diet, as it blends well with smoothies, and provides a desert-like flavor that satisfies most sugar cravings, while supporting overall health.

- ## Bee Pollen

Bee pollen is the food of young bees, and is approximately 40% protein. It contains more amino acids than an equal weight of eggs, or beef. Bee pollen provides almost all the nutrients required by the body, and, therefore, is considered one of nature's most completely nourishing foods.

Bee pollen is an excellent source of vitamin A, and contains other nutrients, such as B-vitamins, magnesium, iron, zinc, and calcium. Moreover, it has powerful antibacterial, antifungal, and antiviral properties. Bee pollen has been used around the world to support the immune system and prevent infections, such as the cold, flu, and seasonal allergies. It further appears to improve endurance and vitality, supports digestive health, reduces inflammation, and helps prevent, and possibly reverse, malnourishment. Considering the high nutrient profile of bee pollen, it can be used as a powerful dietary supplement to naturally boost your nutrient intake.

- **Raw honey**

Like its relative, bee pollen, raw honey is an amazing superfood that has been consumed around the world for centuries. Unlike processed honey, raw honey is not depleted of its incredible nutritional value and health benefits. It contains live enzymes, antioxidants, anti-inflammatory compounds, vitamins, and minerals, making it not only a sweetener, but a great whole food. The list of health benefits of raw honey is long. It contains antibacterial and antifungal properties, causing it to be beneficial in the treatment of cough, burns, and wounds. It is believed to aid poor quality of sleep, by promoting the release of melatonin in the brain. It can also be utilized to promote healthy digestion, prevent and fight infections, provide natural allergy relief, and boost overall immunity. Many people who suffer with seasonal allergies have found local, raw honey to be helpful, because it desensitizes them to the elements in their region that trigger their allergic reactions.

- ## Maca Powder:

Maca is a root vegetable grown in the Peruvian Andes that has been used as a food and medication, in South America for centuries. Besides providing vitamins and minerals, maca powder is known as an energy booster and a powerful adoptogenic plant. Adaptogens are natural compounds in foods that help the body to deal with persistent stress and fatigue, as well as work to regulate hormones. Hence, maca powder may impact PMS, menopausal symptoms, and prostate cancer in men.

As an example, I had a client who was going through menopause and struggling with intensive hot flashes that disrupted her sleep. Within weeks of using the powder, her symptoms were gone, and she was enjoying a good night's sleep again, free of the night sweats.

- ## Ashwagandha Root

Ashwagandha is another powerful adaptogenic plant popular in Ayurvedic medicine, for restoring balance in the body, boosting brain function, and strengthening the immune system. Its botanical name is *Withania somnifera*, and it is known as Indian ginseng. Adaptogenic herbs work within the body to restore balance to the hormonal system, whether levels are high or low.

The adaptogenic benefit of ashwagandha has been notable, for lowering cortisol, improving insulin sensitivity, and leveling thyroid hormones.

One of the things that make weight loss difficult, for many people, is an imbalance of these hormones. Adding ashwagandha to your diet may go a long way toward effectively achieving a weight loss goal. Additionally, this plant has been shown to have powerful anti-cancer properties. In addition to preventing cancer cells from growing, studies have shown that ashwagandha may also be a very useful complement to chemotherapy, when treating existing cancer.

- Acerola cherry powder

Acerola cherries are a powerhouse of antioxidants that protect the body from degenerative diseases and rapid aging. If you wish to increase your vitamin C intake with food, acerola cherries are the answer. A single teaspoon of unripe, acerola cherry powder contains 1,114 mg of vitamin C, which is 1,800% of the recommended daily value, making it one of the best food sources of vitamin C available. This high content of vitamin C, found in acerola cherry powder, makes it a great food for maintaining healthy gums, eyes, and skin. It is also effective at protecting and defending the nervous system, from degenerative diseases, supporting the cardiovascular and respiratory systems, and promoting liver detoxification. Acerola cherry powder is energizing, mood-lifting, and highly useful in strengthening the immune system. The benefit of getting vitamin C, from whole foods, such as acerola cherry powder, instead of in a synthetic form (ascorbic acid), is that the synergetic effect, with the other nutrients in foods you are consuming, makes it more powerful in the body.

- Camu Camu Powder

Camu camu is the second-best food source of vitamin C, with 450 mg per teaspoon, which is 750% of daily values. Therefore, it shares the same health benefits of acerola cherries based on its high Vitamin C content.

- Amla, aka Amalaki or Indian Gooseberry

Amla powder, primarily used in traditional, Indian Ayurvedic medicine, contains a variety of antioxidants and anti-inflammatory compounds that have been shown to promote a healthy body. Today, its numerous health benefits are being recognized in many other parts of the world. This wonder berry may support cardiovascular health, by protecting blood vessels from oxidative damage, as well as lowering LDL cholesterol. Amla fortifies the liver, nourishes the brain, and may improve mental functioning. It also appears to regulate blood sugar, promote healthy skin, and boost the immune system.

- Spirulina

Spirulina is a type of live, blue-green algae found in most lakes and ponds. It is an incredible superfood and among the most nutrient-dense foods found. Spirulina is a concentrated source of complete protein, providing all nine essential amino acids. These algae have been consumed, for thousands of years by the Aztecs in Mexico, and are revered for its high nutrition profile. The health benefits of spirulina extend to various bodily functions, including detoxification, proper immune response, protection from oxidative stress, and anti-inflammatory support. Spirulina may also help the body fight infection, alleviate sinus issues, aid with weight loss, and support a heathy heart and brain.

- Chlorella

Like its cousin spirulina, chlorella is a green algae, dense in nutrients, with many health benefits. Its high level of antioxidants, including Beta-Carotene, help prevent cancer, heart diseases, and other chronic diseases linked to oxidative damage. It is rich in iron, and most components of the B-complex vitamins, including

B12, making it a recommended supplement for vegetarians. Chlorella appears to boost energy, support fat loss, and help alleviate negative effects of radiation and chemotherapy, for people receiving cancer treatments.

Chlorella is one of the richest sources of chlorophyll—the substance that gives plants their green color—and is known as the 'green blood' of plants. This is because chlorophyll is similar in chemical structure to hemoglobin, which allows plants to absorb energy from sunlight. The incredible amount of chlorophyll in chlorella makes it invaluable to the body, as it both nourishes and purifies the blood, kidneys, liver, and bowels. The level of chlorophyll in chlorella, also causes it to act as a natural deodorant, by controlling body odor from the inside out.

Further health benefits include: functioning as a powerful detoxifier of the body, by binding and flushing out heavy metals that hinder absorption of nutrients, and cleansing the body of a wide range of other toxins. Considering that we live in such a toxic environment today, we would all benefit from adding chlorella to our diet. When getting chlorella, make certain to choose 'thin cell wall' or "cracked cell wall" chlorella; it is easier for the body to digest.

- **Chaga Mushroom Powder**

Chaga (Inonotus obliquus) is a medicinal mushroom, a type of fungus which grows on birch trees in Siberia and other cold regions like Alaska and Northern Canada. It has been used in Eastern European folk medicine as a natural remedy for a wide selection of conditions. In Asian culture, chaga mushroom is referred to as the "Mushroom of Immortality" and is frequently used for immune system support to resist and fight infection. Chaga mushroom has gained popularity recently in the West, where its health benefits are now supported by science.

Chaga mushrooms contain large amounts of phytonutrients and immune supporting compounds such as Beta Glycans and polysaccharides which support the body's ability to set up cellular defenses. Another amazing compound found in chaga mushrooms is betulinic acid; it is known to induce apoptosis or cell death and prevent tumors from developing. A number of research articles have confirmed that chaga has exciting anti-tumor potential. Besides strengthening the immune system and preventing tumors from developing, chaga mushrooms may also lower LDL (the "bad" cholesterol) and help with digestion by stimulating digestive bile production which helps break down fatty foods. Because of the incredible immune supporting properties of the chaga mushroom, many experts consider it to be one of the most potent natural foods for auto-immune diseases.

On top of all these health benefits, chaga mushroom is also an adaptogen. As we learned earlier, adaptogens help the body deal with stress by balancing hormones. So, as you can see, this medicinal mushroom is another powerhouse of health benefits you need in your diet; it's so easy to just add it to your smoothie!

Other medicinal mushrooms you can add to your smoothies include Reishi, Maitake, and Shiitake mushrooms.

Noni Fruit Powder

Noni is high in phytochemicals, mainly polyphenols, and flavonoids. Studies have shown that these phytochemicals provide high antioxidant activities, which help reduce the risk of cancer, heart disease and other degenerative diseases.

The noni fruit is referred to as the "queen of health plants" due to its numerous health benefits, and have been used in Ayuvedic and Chinese medicine for thousands of years. Amount these health benefits the noni fruit may support the immune system by increasing the production of T cells. These are like the soldiers of your body immune system that fight invaders, including toxins.

The immunomodulatory effect of noni might also be helpful for people dealing with autoimmune disease.

Noni has anti-inflammatory, analgesic, and anti-cancer effects. Some studies have compared the pain relief effect of noni to some opioid medications such as Tramadol, with great result, yet without the addictive effect. So if you are dealing with pain, including arthritis pain, migraine, and fibromyalgia pain, adding noni to your diet may be helpful. One of the easiest ways is to just add it to your smoothie.

- ## Raw Unrefined Apple Cider Vinegar

Unlike refined and distilled vinegars, commonly found in supermarkets, raw unrefined apple cider vinegar has a murky appearance, yet retains the culture of beneficial bacteria that turns regular apple cider into vinegar. This is like the SCOBY (Symbiotic Culture of Bacteria and Yeast), called a 'mother' in Kombucha making. Raw, unrefined apple cider vinegar is an ancient folk-remedy that boasts that it positively impacts all sorts of health problems. Today, science has proven that apple cider vinegar shows great promise of improving insulin sensitivity and lowering blood sugar responses. For this reason, it can be useful for people with diabetes, or pre-diabetics.

Many believe that raw, unrefined apple cider vinegar also improves blood pressure, balances cholesterol levels, and boosts the body's ability to resist and fight infections. Even if these claims are not documented by science, unrefined apple cider vinegar is rich in bioactive compounds, including acetic acid, good bacteria, and enzymes. These bioactive compounds have shown to be beneficial to our health at different levels. It, therefore, is worth giving raw, unrefined apple cider vinegar a try, by adding it to your smoothies.

Now you know all about my favorite smoothie superfoods! You, however, can add any foods that are high in nutrients, and/or provide desired health benefits, to your drinks. You just need to make sure that taste will blend well, with the other ingredients in your smoothie, and make your taste buds happy. You are in control!

NOTES

Chapter Twelve
Tips for a great Smoothie Experience

❖ ❖ ❖ ❖ ❖ ❖

*T*he basic recipe formula for superfood-smoothies that I proposed in Chapter Nine makes a large batch that would, obviously, not be consumed at one time, but provides enough to be saved for later.

This strategy allows you to prepare once, and reap the benefits twice, or more times, as desired. An advantage of making a large batch is that it allows you to easily meet your daily fruit and vegetable requirements, with the least amount of time.

Thusly, with two cups of green leafy vegetables and two cups of fruit, including the bananas, we have a total of six servings (2 vegetables and 4 fruits). Even if the only fruit you consume a day is in a smoothie, you will have eaten four servings of fruit, meeting experts' recommendation.

After drinking a smoothie, you have three vegetable servings left to meet healthy, dietary guidelines. If you decide to have a salad, or vegetables soup, with your lunch or dinner, and some steamed or stir-fried vegetables with your dinner, you will exceed the remaining three servings of vegetables recommended. Here is how: the vegetable soup gives you at least one serving, and the salad gives you one+ serving, since there is usually at least one cup of greens and probably 1/2 cup of other veggies, such as tomatoes, onion, bell pepper, and cucumber. At dinner, one cup of steamed, roasted, or stir-fry vegetables, will give you two more vegetable servings. Along with your smoothie, that scenario provides a minimum of five vegetable servings for the day. In case you are counting, that's 9-10 fruit and vegetable servings in a day.

See how easy it is to consume the recommended 8-10 servings of fruits and vegetables per day, using my smoothie formula. Imagine trying to achieve that healthy dietary goal, without the smoothie. This is the reason I am so passionate about superfood-smoothie. Remember, however, you don't have to make them every day! Different recipes can be made and conveniently stored in the freezer, for up to seven days. How cool is that?

Here are some tips, for a successful smoothie experience:

1. Put your blender and your recipe collection—including this book—in an accessible place.

2. Household blender trick:

   - Work your recipe gradually, adding ingredients a few at a time. Start with the greens, nuts, and seeds, using the liquid in your recipe to blend until chunks are gone.

   - Then, add the fruit—no more than one cup at a time—until everything is smooth. Processing this way is imperative with a household blender. It doesn't have the power to do the work in one step; this is especially true, if you are using flaxseed, kale, and/or frozen fruit.

3. Do not drink a smoothie too fast. Digestion begins in the mouth, not in the stomach, as you might think. Holding your smoothie in your mouth for a few seconds lets saliva mix with the juice, to aid digestion and allow nutrients to absorb.

4. Keep frozen bananas and pineapple on hand in your freezer. They are the two most commonly used fruits in smoothie recipes. For added convenience, it is also recommended to keep frozen berries, mangos, and peaches on hand, as they are readily available pre-frozen. Adding a frozen-fruit component to your smoothie gives it that cool, refreshing taste, even when making it, predominantly, with fresh fruit. When fruit is in season, or on sale, buy fresh produce and freeze it for later.

5. How to freeze bananas and other peeled fruit:
   - Let bananas ripen well—until they have some brown spots—to increase the sweetness and flavor. Remove the peel and cut into chunks.
   - Next, cover a baking sheet that fits into your freezer, with parchment paper, and align the banana chunks in one layer. Freeze for a few hours, then transfer the frozen chunks, into a freezer bag and return it to the freezer. When processing this way, the banana chunks will remain separated so that you can easily measure with your measuring

cup. This prevents the whole bag of fruit from freezing together like a brick.

- This technique is also necessary for freezing peaches, nectarines, apricots, pineapples, and other peeled fruits. With unpeeled fruit, such as berries, simply make sure the fruit is dry before bagging it to freeze.

6. Frozen-fruit smoothie tips:

- When using mostly frozen fruits, it is best to work in batches of no more than one cup of fruits at the time. This technique makes it easier on your blender, whether it is heavy-duty or a common household type.
- If the smoothie you make is still too icy to drink, let it rest for few minutes at room temperature before drinking. Your smoothie will be more like using fresh fruits, but cold enough to enjoy.
- Also you can defrost all fruit except the bananas (for a few minutes, or overnight in the refrigerator). Slightly defrosting the fruits makes it easier to drink especially on cold winter day.

7. Leafy Green Vegetables:

   - Buy greens weekly to avoid waste.

   - Use a variety of greens in your smoothie recipes. Remember that for the maximum health benefit, your body needs a variety of leafy green vegetables. You can start with spinach and kale, but, as you get more comfortable drinking a smoothie, be sure to experiment with other leafy greens mentioned previously.

8. Nut milk substitute:

   - Soak 1/4 cup of raw nuts, such as cashews, or almonds, overnight, or for few hours. Discard the soaking water, and add the nuts to your recipe, using water to blend. You can also use this method with pumpkin seeds or sunflower seeds. Either way, the result gives your smoothie the same texture and taste as when using nut milk.

9. Make certain to rotate your recipes. I know it is tempting to stick with ones that you really like, but, keep in mind, "Variety is the spice of life;" this is equally true with smoothies. Each fruit, vegetable, and superfood, including

nuts and seeds, has something unique to offer. Therefore, it is critical to make different recipes, so you get the most from nature's bounty.

10. Storing blended smoothies in the refrigerator:
- For maximum freshness, nutrition, and taste, it is best to consume your smoothie within 24 hours. Nevertheless, left-overs will keep, when refrigerated, for up to 48 hours.
- Refrigerate in glass jars (I use 16 oz. Mason jars) with airtight lids, to store for later enjoyment.
- If you want you can add some lemon, or lime juice to help preserve freshness and minimize oxidation.
- Fill the jar all the way to the top, leaving no air gap, then close the jar with an airtight lid.
- Refrigerate your smoothie, in the coldest part of the refrigerator.

11. When ready to drink your refrigerated smoothie, you can add some lemon or lime juice before giving it a good stir, and you will have a fresh tasting smoothie. If frozen ingredients are used in your original smoothie batch, the texture will be slightly different, as your left-overs defrost

in the refrigerator—a little thinner consistency—and ingredients tend to separate.

12. Freeze-ahead ready to blend smoothie prep tricks:

- Do your prep work first, and then freeze individual recipes for up to four weeks, to ensure best quality.
- Wash leafy green vegetables and spin or pat dry.
- Cut fresh fruit into chunks, or use pre-frozen fruit chunks.
- You will need either quart-sized freezer bags, or 32-ounce wide-mouth Mason jars, along with measuring cups, and nametags, if using jars.
- Label the freezer bags, or jars, with the recipe's name and date.
- Measure the fruit first, then the greens, packing them either in bags or jars. When using bags, remove as much air as possible, before sealing them closed. If using jars, pack fruit and greens loosely and firmly screw on the lid. Be sure to leave some air space, to keep them from breaking.
- Store smoothie bags away from foods, with strong odors. Glass jars offer the best odor protection. Either way, frozen ingredients stay fresh, for up to a month.

- To use a frozen smoothie recipe later, thaw an individual bag, or jar, for about an hour. This will allow the ingredients to slide easily out of the container. Then, blend with the other ingredients in your recipe, and voila—a yummy home-made smoothie!

13. Storing blended smoothies in the freezer:
- You can prepare and freeze individual, blended smoothie servings once a week and enjoy a smoothie every day.
- Select recipes and gather the ingredients for a week of smoothies.
- Make the smoothies and pour individual smoothie servings into freezer-safe jars, such as 16 oz. wide-mouth Mason jars, leaving some space at the top, to prevent the jar from breaking, as the contents expand.
- Label the jars with recipe names and dates.
- Safely store your smoothies in the freezer, for up to seven days.
- Each day, select the smoothies you would like to drink the next day, and place in the refrigerator overnight. When ready to drink, if it is still too frozen to drink, set the jar on the counter and let it thaw for about an hour

or so. After thawing your smoothie, give it a couple of good shakes, to remix the ingredients, and enjoy. You can also add some lemon or lime juice before shaking.

14. Remember, if you are dealing with a chronic health condition, and would like to benefit from the health benefits of fruits and vegetables, it will be helpful to consume the whole smoothie from one recipe. You can divide it into two or three daily servings.

Now that you have these tips and tricks up your sleeve, see how simple it is to have a superfood-smoothie every day, and improve your health and vitality, at the same time.

Chapter Thirteen
Blending vs. Juicing

❖❖❖❖❖❖

*I*t is well established that increasing your intake of fruits and vegetables is critical to attaining optimal health and vitality. The more fruits and vegetables you consume, the greater the benefits! As we mentioned in previous chapters, however, it is difficult for most people to consume the recommended 8-10 servings per day. Fortunately, blending fruit and vegetables into smoothies, or processing them into juices, are easy ways to reach your nutritional goals. Both blending and juicing have become extremely popular these days, but you may be wondering what the difference is.

Blending is a process in which a blender pulverizes the whole product, along with added liquid, to create a relatively thick drink known as a smoothie. Juicing, on the other hand, utilizes a machine (a juicer) to extract the water, and most of the nutrients, from produce, leaving behind the pulp, or fiber, as waste. This

157

procedure results in a watery drink, with a high concentration of nutrients.

You may be thinking, "But, I thought fiber was good for you." You are right, fiber is good for you. It is a form of carbohydrate that is not easily digested by the digestive system. Fiber is primarily found in plant foods, including vegetables, fruits, legumes, whole grains, nuts, and seeds, and appears in two forms—soluble fiber and insoluble fiber. The solubility of fiber refers to its ability to dissolve in water. Both types of fiber serve important functions within the body, and provide many health benefits. They aid in balancing blood sugar, regulating bowel movements, lowering LDL cholesterol, and promoting overall intestinal health, by enhancing the good bacteria in the gut. Fiber also promotes satiety, which makes you feel full for a longer period, after eating. This is particularly beneficial in achieving and maintaining a healthy weight.

Knowing that the juicing process removes fiber, you might think that juicing may not be as healthy as smoothies. The good news is that it is primarily the insoluble fiber that is left out. Most of the soluble fiber is incorporated into the juice, along with the water and nutrients, from the fruits and vegetables. As a result, the benefit from fiber, in the juices, is derived from the soluble fiber.

Insoluble fiber is important, however, because it does make you feel full and promotes the movement of material through the digestive tract, evidenced in increased stool bulk, thus preventing constipation. Considering that juicing is not the only component of your diet, you will consume enough insoluble fiber, from the whole foods you eat, especially if you include smoothies as well.

Thusly, juicing is a great addition to a healthy diet, since it allows you to consume a concentrated amount, and variety, of vitamins, minerals, enzymes, and phytochemicals. When it comes to blending vs juicing, either process helps to increase your fruit and vegetable intake, thus boosting your health. Both techniques have some pros and some cons, and, in certain circumstances, one may be a better choice than the other, as you can see in the table below.

Criteria	Smoothie (Blending)	Juice (Juicing)
Cost	Less up-front investment since a household blender can do the job at a lower cost; does not require as much produce as with juicing.	More up-front investment as a juicer is required; more ongoing cost, since a greater volume of produce is used to make a glass of juice.

Waste	There is no waste with blending— what is put in the blender is what you consume.	Juicing involves some waste; insoluble fiber and some nutrients might be removed.
Satiety	Very satiating as it is loaded with fiber. Added protein makes it a complete meal replacement.	Though nutrient-dense, it is not satisfying enough to be a complete meal replacement.
Contraindications	High fiber content can be an issue for people with digestive disorders, such as IBS, Crohn's disease and other inflammatory bowel diseases.	Lack of insoluble fiber makes it easier on the digestive system; a better choice for people with IBS, Crohn's disease and other inflammatory bowel diseases.
Effect on blood sugar	High amount of fiber and added protein may slow down digestion and absorption of nutrients; provides a more sustainable energy level and blood sugar control.	Lack of insoluble fiber speeds up digestion and absorption of nutrients, providing quick energy; can lead to blood sugar spikes

Tolerance during sickness	For people seriously ill, or recovering from sickness or surgery, it may be harder to drink a smoothie, and more difficult for a weak body to digest and absorb the nutrients.	For people seriously ill, or recovering from sickness, it is easier to drink a juice, and easier for a weak body to digest and absorb the nutrients.
Convenience	Blending takes less time and is more convenient; frozen fruits can be used. Also, less clean-up involved with smoothies.	Juicing is more time consuming and less convenient; fresh produce is needed for preparation. More clean-up is also involved.

Conclusion

Juicing and blending are both great ways to include a lot of produce, and greater variety, in your diet. With a few exceptions, most people can benefit from these practices; therefore, it is worth trying them both! Considering that blending smoothies requires less investment than juicing, and preparation is more convenient, it may be better to start with it—especially if both time and budget are limited. Later, when having a superfood-smoothie on a regular basis has become a habit, add something else—like juicing.

Chapter Fourteen
Juicing 101

❖❖❖❖❖❖

$\mathcal{J}$uicing is mostly about increasing your intake of vegetable. To make vegetable juice more palatable, a little bit of fruit is added, for a touch of sweetness. Too much fruit added to the juice, however, will cause sugars to rapidly absorb into the bloodstream. This can trigger a spike in blood sugar and contribute to insulin resistance, Type 2 diabetes, and/or weight gain.

Benefits of juicing, when done properly:

- Hydrates the body
- Provides a concentrated amount and variety of nutrients to nourish the body
- Boosts the immune system
- Boosts energy and mental clarity
- Supports detoxification

- Supports healing and repair
- Easy way to include a variety of vegetables to kid's diet, especially when they are picky eaters.

Equipment needed for juicing:

To properly juice vegetables, a 'juicer', a knife, a cutting board, and citrus press are necessary tools for prepping your produce. Glass bottles, or jars, with airtight lids (12-18 ounces), are best used for storing purposes.

Buying a good juicer can be a challenging process, since prices vary widely—from less than $100 to more than $1,000 per appliance. What you need to know is that there are different types of equipment—the most common ones are centrifugal and masticating juicers.

Centrifugal juicers are the most popular, as they are the ones you see most, in TV advertisements or department stores. They operate by shredding ingredients, with a rapidly spinning disk of blades, and then filtering them, through a very fine strainer. They do tend to be less expensive than masticating juicers, and are easier to use and clean. On the downside, these machines extract a little less juice, especially from leafy green vegetables and grasses. Furthermore, the juice from a centrifugal juicer may be more prone to oxidization, because of the high friction generated, during the process. Some people are concerned about the speed required, in the spinning process, and worry that it might generate heat that could destroy the enzymes in the juice. The truth is that the heat produced is barely detectible and not enough to damage the enzymes. The juice, from a centrifugal juicer, is as nutritious as that from a masticating juicer. Breville is a good brand that is affordable, and yet performs well and is durable. The JE98XL model is the most popular, and probably the best value for the money (about $140). If you can afford a higher model like a Breville BJE430SIL (about $180), however, that is better.

Masticating juicers operate by first crushing and then pressing fruit and vegetables, for the highest quality yield. This process is done slowly, so there is not a lot of friction generated. For this reason, these juicers are also known as 'cold-press' juicers. These appliances extract more juice than its centrifugal counterpart, and the juice tends to retain its quality longer. Nevertheless, this type of juicer cannot handle whole pieces of fruit or vegetables as well. They generally come with chutes that are quite narrow, and allow only small amounts to be processed at a time. This means that more prep work is required—to chop and cut up the ingredients. This is necessary before inserting them into the unit. Most centrifugal juicers have a wider chute for adding food, which makes them more time efficient.

Consequently, a masticating juicer does not produce juice as quickly, as the centrifugal type. Masticating juicers cost more, and it is extremely difficult to find a good one priced at less than $250—many units sell for over $500. Omega J8004 Nutrition Center is a good model, costing approximately $250. To its credit, it also does more than juice. It can be used to make fresh frozen desserts, natural baby food, nut butters, and nut milk.

When it comes to how long these super juices can last in the refrigerator, it does not matter whether the juice was made with a centrifugal or mastication juicer. After a few days in the refrigerator, the taste and quality of the juice will be adversely affected, regardless of machine. If you are not able to make juice every day, there are some tips that will allow you to extend its life. You will find them at the end of this chapter.

Common produce used for juicing:

Such greens as kale and spinach are not the primary vegetables in my juices. Instead, they are the stars of my superfood-smoothies. For juicing purposes, cabbage (especially red cabbage) is a major player. The reason being that cabbage is frequently overlooked in most daily diets, even though it contains a wealth of important nutrients and disease-fighting phytonutrients. It comes in many varieties—savoy, spring green, green, red, and white cabbage, which is most commonly found in grocery stores. Cabbage juice has been used in many cultures, around the world, to heal stomach ulcers and affect digestive disorders such as irritable bowel syndrome (IBS), Crohn's disease, and other inflammatory bowel diseases. As you may recall, from an earlier chapter, cabbage is part of the cruciferous vegetables, along with kale and collard greens. Hence, they share many of the same health benefits, as cancer prevention and detoxification. It also helps to lower the LDL cholesterol levels in blood, which can build up in arteries and cause heart disease. Cabbage further contains the highest number of antioxidants found in cruciferous vegetables.

Besides these healing properties, cabbage is a powerhouse of nutrients, with an incredible amount of vitamins C and K. Their high content of vitamin C explains why cabbages are such an obvious antioxidant that supports the immune system, by stimulating the activity of white blood cells. Additionally, vitamin

K boosts a specific protein required to maintain bone calcium, reducing the risk of osteoporosis. Cabbage is, also, an excellent source of the B-complex vitamins known to boost energy. Rich in manganese, iron, magnesium, phosphorus, calcium for strong bones, and potassium, for supporting a healthy heart rate and blood pressure, this vegetable is a must in any diet.

Although all cabbages share these properties, red cabbage has something the others do not possess: the polyphenol anthocyanin. The red/purple color of red cabbage is reflective of anthocyanin—a highly praised antioxidant found in berries and red wine that has been linked to cardiovascular and brain health. It has been found to have more anthocyanins than either red wine or certain berries, is considered a brain food, because of the high level of anthocyanins that influence mental functioning and concentration, and prevents nerve damage, improving a defense against degenerative brain diseases, such as Alzheimer's.

Now you see why I consider cabbage to be the star in my vegetable juices. Because of its high, water content, it is an excellent vegetable to juice; it is also very affordable and in season year-round. Cabbage is part of the "Clean 15" list, from the Environmental Working Group's Guide to Pesticides in Produce— noted as one of the vegetables with the lowest amount of pesticide residue. For this reason, you do not need to buy organic cabbage.

Although I choose to make cabbage, especially red cabbage, the principal vegetable in my juice, it does not mean I never juice other greens—especially when they are in season and/or on sale. As mentioned before, I like to utilize vegetables that I am less likely to use in my smoothies; i.e. mustard greens, dandelion greens, and turnip greens.

Other vegetables to use in juices:

- **Carrots** – Loaded with beta carotene, a precursor to vitamin A that acts as an antioxidant.
- **Celery** – High in electrolytes and antioxidants, with very low calories; acts as diuretic, and supports the digestive tract. Also promotes healthy weight control.
- **Cucumbers** – High in electrolytes and antioxidants; provides many vitamins and minerals, with low calorie count. Cucumbers also promote healthy weight control.
- **Beets** – Loaded with antioxidants and anti-inflammatory compounds. Promote kidney health, and support detoxification and healthy blood pressure.

- **Fennel bulb** – High in antioxidants, vitamin C, potassium, and other nutrients. Supports a healthy blood pressure, due to the high amount of potassium.

- **Sweet potatoes** – Powerhouse of antioxidants and anti-inflammatory phytonutrients; exceptionally high in beta carotene (in yellow sweet potatoes) and anthocyanins— the same nutrients found in berries and red wine (in purple sweet potatoes).

- **Tomatoes** – Provide a wide range of nutrients and exceptionally high in lycopene, a phytonutrient linked to cardiovascular health and prevention of prostate cancer.

Besides their health benefits, these vegetables are great for juicing, because they have a high water content, which results in more juice and less waste. Some of them also bring a touch of sweetness to the juice (carrots, sweet potatoes, and beets)

Fruits to use in juices:

As we mentioned earlier, the fruits used in juicing are there primarily to provide a bit of sweetness to the vegetable juice. Therefore, look for fruit that is sweet, high in water content, available all year- round, and low in cost. Apples meet these criteria, and are the primary fruit in my juices. Other choices are lemons, or lime, because their tartness helps to offset the strong taste of some vegetables. The vitamin C in these fruit, also acts as a food preservative, by reducing the risk of oxidation when exposed to oxygen.

Pears, pineapple, and melons are also good choices, when they are in season. They are sweet, filled with liquid, and add extra flavor to any juice.

It is important to peel citrus fruits before juicing, if you don't want the juice to taste bitter. I prefer using a citrus press, to add citrus fruit to my juice.

Herbs and spices

All herbs and spices are high in antioxidants, as well as additional bioactive compounds that promote health, at different levels in the body; juicing is a great way to add them to your diet. For me, herbs work better with juicing than adding them to my smoothies. Besides their health benefits, herbs and spices also add flavor. I often use:

- **Mint** - supports digestion and offers anti-inflammatory benefits. Adds a delightful flavor to the juice.
- **Cilantro and parsley** - great for the liver, supports proper detoxification. Cilantro also has antimicrobial properties.

- **Basil** - provides antimicrobial and anti-inflammatory benefits.

- **Ginger and Turmeric** – well known for their anti-inflammatory and analgesic (pain reducing) benefits. Ginger gives a slight spicy kick to the drink, depending on how much you use. Also helps offset the strong taste of some vegetables, whether it is cabbage or leafy greens, such as kale. For this reason, ginger is a common ingredient in my juices.

Besides these herbs and spices, you can also use any others that you enjoy, or are easily available. Just make sure the flavor blends well, with the other ingredients in your recipe.

Nathalie's Juice Recipe Formula:

You can juice any vegetable you want, as long as it has enough water to be processed. However, to make a truly good juice, it must contain the following:

- Something sweet
- Something tart
- Something with a high yield, and
- Something flavorful and/or spicy (optional)

As indicated above, fruits, such as apples, pears, pineapple, and melons will provide sweetness to your vegetable juice. Lemons, lime, and pineapple offer tartness. Cucumbers, celery, carrots, beets, sweet potatoes, and cabbage are high yield vegetables. When juicing leafy greens, a fruit is needed for sweetness, as well as another high yield vegetable, to fill a glass. Ginger, can then be added for a spicy kick; cilantro, parsley, mint, or basil add additional flavor.

When choosing a food from each category, consider how it will taste with the other ingredients in your recipe, and make certain the combination seems pleasing to your taste buds. Remember, juicing is like cooking; you can always adjust the ingredients, if you feel something more, or less, is needed. When not sure what to adjust, add a piece of ginger, or more lemon; this will bring freshness to the drink.

Consider color

It is important to remember that the way food looks affects our perception of the way it will taste. Therefore, color adds interest to any food. Bright colors, such as green, orange, and red, or purple, are more appealing than pale ones, like gray or brown. Thusly, when preparing a juice, decide the color you would like, and then select fruits and vegetables that will provide that color.

Common colors of juices, and the primary produce to achieve it:

- **Green juice:** leafy greens (kale, collard greens, mustard greens, turnip greens, etc.), celery, and cucumber
- **Orange juice:** carrots, sweet potatoes, cantaloupe, and turmeric
- **Red/purple:** beets, red cabbage, watermelon, and tomatoes

To concoct your own recipe, follow the rules above, and you will create a juice that is both appealing to the eye and pleasant to the taste buds.

Tips for a successful juicing experience:

- Remember that with juicing, the emphasis is on vegetables. Always use more vegetables than fruits.

- It is best to drink juice immediately, whenever possible. For most people, it is not easy to make juice daily. For that reason, make a large batch and keep it for later. To do this, fill a glass jar, or bottle, to the top, close it tightly, and refrigerate it, for a maximum of 24 hours. To save longer, freeze it.

- To safely freeze your juice, make several recipes, and immediately freeze in glass bottles, or jars (I use 8 or 16 oz. Mason jar). Do not fill them completely, as, at least one inch of space is needed for expansion, so the container does not break when freezing. Defrost one serving, in the refrigerator overnight; the next day, give it a good shake and enjoy your juice.

- Always add lemon, or lime, to your juice. This is critical, not only for the flavor, but, also, because the high level of vitamin C acts as a preservative and antioxidant.

- Do not gulp juice too fast. Holding it, in the mouth for few seconds, allows saliva to mix with the juice, facilitating better digestion and absorption of nutrients.

- For best absorption, if possible, drink juice on an empty stomach. The primary benefit of juicing is that it provides an abundance of nutrients that are easily absorbed by the body. This is the consequence of little fiber in the mix. Drinking juice on a full stomach nullifies this benefit. It is advised to drink your juice 20-30 minutes, before a meal, or two hours after. I like to drink my vegetable juice in the morning before breakfast, or mid-day after lunch.

- Rotate vegetables on a regular basis. In the health food community, it is said, "Make sure to eat the rainbow." The colors of different vegetables—red, green, blue/purple, and yellow/orange—represent different types of phytonutrients. Therefore, by including all these colors, you can be assured of a variety of phytonutrients.

- Do not only focus on what you like best. Pungent vegetables, such as cabbage, onions, leeks, mustard greens, dandelion, and arugula, often have specific health benefits linked to their less pleasant taste. By including these stronger, flavored vegetables, you will reap many specific, health benefits useful to the body.

- Make certain to include red cabbage in your juicing habits—perhaps even making it the star. As mentioned earlier, this is a powerhouse vegetable.

- Always clean your juicer immediately after using. Leaving it to clean later will only require more time and effort. If immediate washing is not possible, at least leave it to soak in soapy water, until you have time.

NOTES

Chapter Fifteen
Superfoods and Their Benefits

❖❖❖❖❖❖

*T*his recap is intended to help you select superfoods for your smoothies that are tailored to meet your specific health needs. To begin with, choose few superfoods that you would like to try, and are easily available. Use them consistently for at least four to eight weeks. Some results may be noticeable, within a few days; others will take longer, to work their magic. Give them a good effort, however, before expecting full results.

Keep in mind that the impact of superfoods is not limited to only the health benefits mentioned below. They often work in a synergistic way, with other foods you consume, to nourish and heal your body at different levels.

Important note: many of these superfoods have powerful pharmaceutical effects that could interact with medications you are taking. For that reason, always check with your doctor, before beginning this dietary regimen.

As an example, if you are taking Metformin for diabetes, and add cinnamon, turmeric, or black seed to your diet, the additions could double the effect of your medication and result in too low a blood sugar. Therefore, if you are on any medications, have your doctor review this list and determine, if there are any potential interactions that would be harmful to your health. As time passes, keep him informed of any changes you experience. He can then either adjust, or cancel, medications as indicated. Consuming superfoods on a regular basis can regulate the body and frequently even reduce the need for medications altogether. That is the power of plant foods!

Beneficial effects and the superfoods that produce them:

- ## Blood Pressure/Heart and brain Health
    - o Unsulfured blackstrap molasses
    - o Flaxseeds
    - o Chia seeds
    - o Hemp seeds
    - o Amla

- Tumrmeric
- Noni
- Ginger
- Acai berries
- Goji berries
- Ashwagandha
- Acerola cherry
- Camu camu
- Black seeds
- Nuts and seeds
- Raw cacao powder
- Collagen hydrolysate
- Whey protein
- Matcha green tea
- Chaga mushrooms

- **Blood Sugar Control**
  - Cinnamon
  - Turmeric
  - Moringa
  - Goji Berry
  - Apple cider vinegar
  - Blackstrap molasses
  - Amla

- Black seeds
- Nuts and seeds
- Collagen hydrolysate
- Whey protein Isolate
- Chaga mushrooms

- **Cholesterol Regulation**
  - Amla
  - Turmeric
  - Unsulfured blackstrap molasses
  - Black seeds
  - Flaxseed
  - Chia seeds
  - Hemp seeds
  - Goji berries
  - Nuts and seeds
  - Raw cacao powder
  - Cinnamon
  - Ginger
  - Matcha green tea
  - Chaga mushroom

- **Detoxification**
  - Chlorella
  - Spurilina

- Moringa
- Acerola cherry
- Camu camu
- Barley grass
- Wheat grass
- Amla
- Black seeds
- Chaga mushrooms

- **Energy Booster**
  - Maca
  - Moringa
  - Ashwagandha
  - Acerola cherries
  - Camu camu
  - Chlorella
  - Spirulina
  - Matcha green tea
  - Collagen hydrolysate
  - Whey protein

- **Hormone Support**
  - Ashwagandha
  - Maca
  - Flaxseed

- Chia seeds
- Hemp seeds
- Nuts and seeds
- Chaga mushrooms

- **Immune System Support**
  - Black seeds
  - Chaga mushrooms
  - Noni
  - Acerola cherry
  - Camu camu
  - Goji berry
  - Amla
  - Chlorella
  - Spirulina
  - Bee pollen
  - Raw honey
  - Nuts and seeds

- **Anti-inflammatory/Pain relief**
  - Turmeric
  - Ginger
  - Black seeds
  - Noni
  - Amla

- Chia seeds
- Hemp seeds
- Flaxseeds
- Collagen hydrolysate
- Chaga mushrooms

- **Skin Health**
  - Collagen Hydrolysate
  - Acerola cherries
  - Camu camu
  - Amla
  - Black seeds
  - Nuts

Best food source of some nutrients

Nutrients	Food Source
Vitamin A	Chlorella, Sweet potatoes, carrots, greens, winter squash
Vitamin C	Acerola cherry, camu camu, Papaya, bell peppers, broccoli, Brussels sprouts, strawberries, pineapple, oranges, kiwi, cantaloupe, cauliflower
Vitamin D	Shiitake mushrooms, Cow's milk
Vitamin E	Sunflower seeds, almonds, spinach, Swiss chard, avocado, spinach, turnip greens, beet greens, mustard greens
Folate	Lentils, beans, spinach, turnip greens, broccoli
Iron	Chlorella, blackstrap molasses, edamame, lentils, moringa, spinach, sesame seeds, beans, Swiss chard, tofu
Calcium	Tofu, blackstrap molasses, sesame seeds, yogurt, turnip greens, mustard greens, collard greens, spinach, cottage cheese, beet greens, cow's milk
Magnesium	Blackstrap molasses, pumpkin seeds, spinach, Swiss chard, edamame, sesame seeds, beans, cashew, sunflower seeds

Potassium	Blackstrap molasses, leafy greens (higher in beet greens and Swiss chard), lima beans, sweet potatoes, edamame, avocado, pinto beans, lentils, banana, kiwi
Zinc	Pumpkin seeds, sesame seeds, lentils, garbanzo beans, cashew
Fiber	All plant foods

NOTES

Chapter Sixteen
Conclusion

❖❖❖❖❖❖

*A*s we have discussed, the root cause, of most chronic conditions affecting people today, is poor diet. Face it! The American standard diet of heavily processed foods is mostly devoid of adequate nutrition, leaving both our bodies and minds malnourished.

Fighting conditions like obesity, Type 2 diabetes, high blood pressure, heart diseases, cancers, and autoimmune diseases is an up-hill battle, considering today's diets. Unless we go "back to the basics," by again focusing on consuming a variety of plant foods, we are doomed to becoming an increasingly unhealthy nation.

There is healing power in nature, and the challenge is to bring it to our bodies, in a convenient way. With our western way of eating, it is almost impossible to meet the recommended 8-10 servings of fruits and vegetables per day that have been linked to improving, or even reversing, some chronic diseases. For this reason, I have become passionate about finding a way to achieve this goal. That way has been to create superfood-smoothies and juices that provide the nutrition the body requires to be healthy and overflowing with vitality. These superfood-smoothies and juices—natural multi-vitamin drinks—can be quick, easy, affordable, and nutritious answers to the health crisis of our society.

If you are sick and tired of being sick and tired, get actively involved in taking back your health, by making superfood-smoothies and/or vegetable juices part of your daily, mealtime routine. It may be a little challenging at first, but following the tips shared in this book can make your experience easy and pleasantly satisfying. Taking multi-vitamin pills may seem easier, but nothing can replace the synergistic effects of nutrients gotten directly from nature. Remember, most good things in life come with some sacrifice, and your body will thank you for your effort!

In the next sections of this book, you will find recipes, and notes, on making some of my favorite superfood-smoothies and vegetable juices. To this point I have described the "why" and "what" of ingredients desperately needed by the body, and now I am excited to share the "how" to making this a reality. It can be fun, affordable, and possible to enhance your health, vitality, and quality of life, by adding these superfood supplements to your dietary regimen.

Just remember, when it comes to consuming more plant foods, like fruits and vegetables, "If you can't eat them, drink them!"

Note: You can make other varieties of this recipe by replacing the blueberries with strawberries, raspberries, blackberries, or mix berries. Considering the critical role of berries on our health, this berry base recipe should be your most common recipe.

Nathalie's Smoothie Favorites

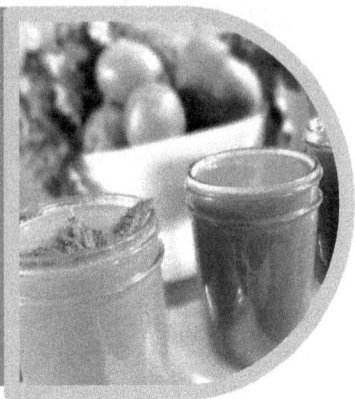

Blue-Pineapple Smoothie

1 cup blueberries

½ cup pineapple

½ cup frozen banana chunks or 1 medium banana

1 cup spinach

1 cup kale

1 tablespoon flaxseed

1 scoop whey protein isolate or ½ cup non-fat, plain Greek yogurt

2 cups milk or water

1 tablespoons raw honey, blackstrap molasses, or 2 soft dates (optional)

Tropical Turmeric Blast (Anti-inflammatory)

1½ cup tropical mix fruits (mango, papaya, pineapple)

½ cup frozen banana chunks or 1 medium banana

½ a small lemon, juiced

2 cups mix greens

1 scoop collagen hydrolysate or whey protein isolate

½ inch fresh ginger (or more)

1-inch turmeric root or 1 tsp turmeric powder

Pinch of black pepper

½ cup boxed coconut milk (I use "So Delicious" brand. You can find it in baking aisle at Walmart)

1½ cups coconut water

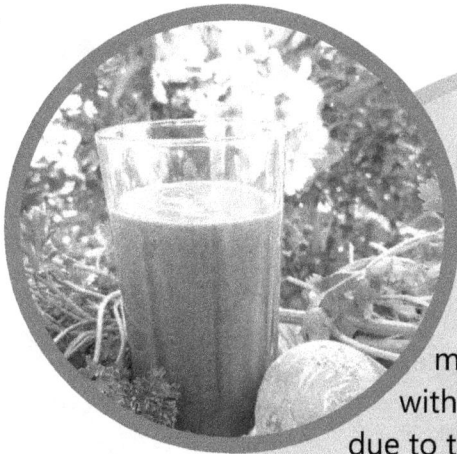

Note: you can also Use 1 cup of mango or papaya, and ½ cup pineapple instead of the mix fruits. This smoothie may be helpful when dealing with pain or menstrual cramps, due to the anti-inflammatory effect of turmeric and ginger.

Sweet Pea Delight

½ cup frozen sweet peas

1 cup mango

1 cup pineapple

1 cup spinach

½ cup frozen sweet peas

½ small avocados

1 teaspoon pure vanilla extract

2 cups milk

Note: Add some water if smoothie is too thick

Strawberry-Kiwi Passion

1 cup strawberries

3-4 kiwis (pealed)

½ cup frozen banana or 1 small banana

2 cups mix greens

1 tablespoon chia seed

1 scoop whey protein isolate

2 cups milk or water

1-2 tablespoons raw honey

Peanut Butter-Fruit Smoothie

1 ½ cup mix fruits (peach, strawberry, mango, pineapple)

½ cup frozen banana chunks or 1 medium banana

2-3 tablespoons peanut powder

2 cups baby mix greens

1 scoop whey protein isolate

1 tablespoon flaxseed

2 cups milk

Kiwi-Honeydew Bliss

2 kiwis

1 cup honey dew

1 cups pineapple

1 cup Bok choy

1 cup spinach

1 scoop whey protein isolate

½ small avocados

2 cups milk

Green Mango-Pineapple Surprise

1 cup mango

½ cup pineapple

½ cup frozen banana chunks or 1 medium banana

1 cup collard green

1 cup spinach

3 tablespoons hemp seeds

2 cups milk

Pomegranate-Berry Smoothie

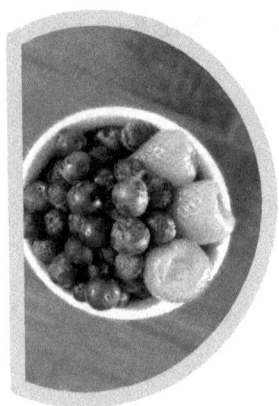

1 cup mixed berries

½ cup pineapple

1 cup Swiss chard

1 cup spinach

½ avocados

2 cups pomegranate juice

1-2 tablespoons raw honey

Orange Ginger-Peach Drink

1 cup peaches

½ cup carrot, chopped

2 cups orange juice (not from concentrate)

½ inch ginger

2 cups spinach

1 scoop whey protein isolate or collagen hydrolysate

1 tablespoon chia seeds

½ a small lemon, juiced

Note: For another variety, use mango, nectarine, or apricot instead of

Raspberry-Chocolate Blast

1 cup raspberries

½ cup pineapple

½ cup frozen banana or 1 medium banana

2 cups baby, mixed greens

½ cup non-fat, Greek yogurt, plain

2 tablespoons raw cacao powder

2 cups milk

1 tablespoon raw honey

1 tablespoon blackstrap molasses

Note: May also use strawberries or cherries instead of

Nectarine-Almond Butter Smoothie

1 cup nectarine

½ cup pineapple

½ cup frozen banana chunks or 1 medium banana

2 cups spinach

1-2 tablespoons almond butter

1 scoop whey protein Isolate

2 cups milk

Peachy-Pineapple Delight

1 cup peach, chopped

1 cup pineapple

2 cups mix greens

¼ cup cashew

1 scoop whey protein isolate

2 cups water or milk

Pineapple-Pear Ginger Blast

1 cup pineapple

2 ripe pears, seeded, chopped

2 cups spinach

½ a small avocado

4 Brazil nuts

½ inch fresh ginger

Juice of ½ a small lemon

2 cups milk

Cherry-Cranberry Creamy Surprise

1 ½ cups frozen cherries, pitted

1 cup Swiss chard or beet greens

1 cup spinach

1 cup 100% cranberry juice

½ cup low-fat cottage cheese

4 walnuts

2 tablespoon sunflower seeds

1 cup milk

Pomegranate-Beet Smoothie

1 medium beet, cooked and pealed

or 2 tablespoons beet powder

1 cup beet greens

1 cup pineapple

1 cup spinach

Note: Make sure the beets are cooked and soft.

3 tablespoons hemp seeds

1 cup 100% pomegranate juice

1 cup milk

Creamy Blackberry-Pomegranate Surprise

1 cup blackberries

2 cups spinach

6 oz. silk tofu

1 tablespoon chia seeds

1 cup 100% pomegranate juice

1 cup milk

Note: May also use cherries instead of blackberries for another variety of the recipe.

Creamy Pina Colada Cooly

1 ½ cup pineapple

½ cup mango, or peach, or nectarine

2 cups spinach

6-8 oz. silken tofu

½ cups boxed coconut milk (look for "so Delicious" in the baking aisle at Walmart)

1½ cups coconut water

Watermelon-Berry Blast

1½ cups raspberry

2 cups watermelon chunks

2 cups mix baby greens

1 tablespoon chia seeds

½ cup Greek yogurt, plain, non-fat

1 cup milk

2 tablespoons raw honey or two soft dates

Note: May also use 1½ cup of any berry, or mixed berries

Turmeric delight with Carrot and orange

1 cup carrot

2 cups orange juice (not from concentrate)

½ cup frozen banana or 1 medium banana

1 cup spinach

3 tablespoons hemp seeds

1 inch ginger root

2 inches turmeric root, or 1 teaspoon turmeric powder

½ a small lemon, juiced

Cherry-Chocolate Breakfast

1 cup cherries

½ cup pineapple

½ cup frozen banana chunks or 1 medium banana

2 cups mixed baby greens

½ cup rolled oats

2 tablespoons cacao powder

1 tablespoon almond butter

2 tablespoons raw honey

2 cups milk

Grape and berry delight

2 cups spinach

1 cup grapes

1 cup mix berries

1 cup cranberry juice

1 cup water

¼ cup pumpkin seeds, presoaked

1 scoop whey protein isolate or ½ cup Greek yogurt, plain

1-2 Tablespoons blackstrap molasses or raw honey

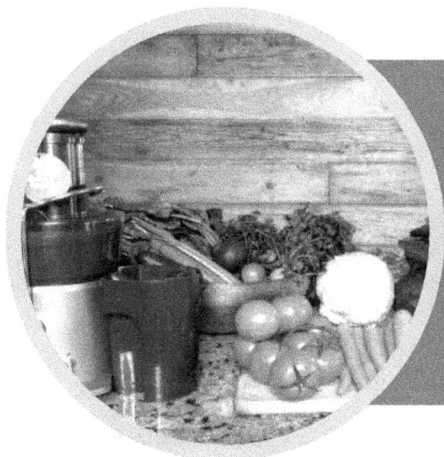

Nathalie's Juicing Favorites

Carrot and Orange Blast

5-6 medium carrots

2 medium juicy oranges, peeled

1-inch ginger root

½ a small lemon, juiced

Note: May also use 100%, not from concentrate orange juice.

Detox Beet Juice

1 medium beet

1 medium apple

1 medium cucumber

1 inch of fresh ginger root

1 handful of parsley

1 handful of cilantro

½ a small lemon, juiced

Note: May also use 4 large celery stalks instead of the cucumber and pears instead of apples.

Anti-Inflammatory Turmeric Juice

2 medium sweet potatoes

2 medium carrots

1 medium apple

1-inch ginger

2 inches turmeric root,

or 1 teaspoon turmeric

powder

½ a small lemon, juiced

Note: If using turmeric powder, add it to the juice. May be helpful when dealing with pain or menstrual cramps, due to the anti-inflammatory effect of turmeric and ginger.

Minty Tomato-Watermelon Juice

2 large tomatoes on the vine

¼ of a small seedless watermelon

6 large mint leaves

½ a lime, juiced

Note: May also add ½ inch ginger for another variety

Green Detox Cooler

1 bunch of kale

2 large celery stalks

1 medium cucumber

1 medium green apple

1-inch ginger root

½ a small lemon, juiced

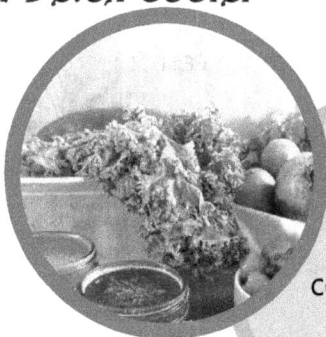

Note: May also use collard or turnip greens.

Super Green Detox Cooler

1 bunch mustard greens

1 medium cucumber

1 medium green apple

1 handful parsley

1 handful cilantro

1 lime, juiced

Note: This juice may have a somewhat unpleasant, peppery taste from the mustard greens. Not recommended for new juicers.

Carrot Juice Blast

5-6 medium carrots

1 apple

1-inch ginger root

1 small lemon, juiced

Spicy Tomato Surprise

3 large tomatoes on the vine

1 medium red apple

1 medium jalapeno (remove half of the seeds for a medium taste or more, for mild taste)

½ a lime, juiced

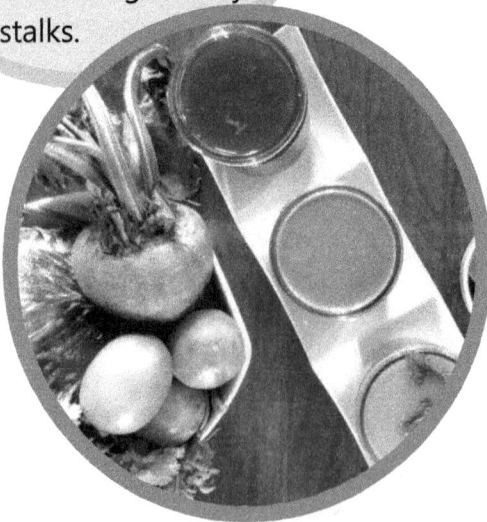

Note: May also add ¼ teaspoon of cayenne paper to the juice, as a substitute to jalapeno. For another variety, use only 2 tomatoes, with 2 large celery stalks.

Red Cabbage Delight

1/2 small red cabbage

1 medium beet

1 medium apple

1-inch ginger root

½ a small lemon, juiced

Note: May also use green cabbage.

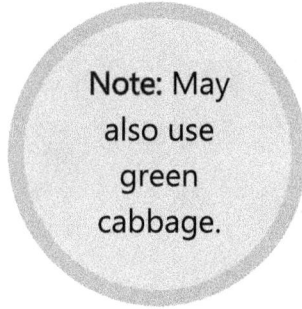

Red Cabbage-Watermelon Delight

½ small red cabbages

¼ a small seedless watermelon

1 inch ginger root

1 small lemon, juiced

NOTES

10-day Reset Plan to Kick-Start Weight loss and Boost your Health

The purpose of this eating plan is to give you a starting point to make superfood-smoothies part of your diet, and experience some of the health benefits of whole foods plant-based diet. During this eating plan all the junk is left out, high carbohydrate foods are cut down and the focus is more on non-starchy vegetable which are higher in phytochemicals and lower in calories. This will not only provide your body with the tool it needs to promote health, but it will also support weight loss due to lower calories meals, yet higher nutrients. It is not a plan to follow for a long period of time. After the 10 days, if you need help implementing a healthy eating lifestyle, contact me for a customized strategy.

You might feel tired the first three days on this plan, this is normal, as your body is adjusting to the change. However, you are expected to feel better after that. If you are still not feeling well, then the plan is probably not good for you, it is then recommended to stop it immediately.

Note: *Please check with your doctor before starting this eating plan to make sure it is safe for you, especially if you are on medication. This plan is not for you if you are pregnant or breastfeeding; or you have IBS or other gastrointestinal disorders.*

Daily plan:

Upon waking up: drink one cup of warm water with the juice of half a lemon. Along with other health benefits, this drink stimulates a bowel movement and cleanses the colon.

Breakfast: Superfood-Smoothie. Drink enough smoothie to feel satiated, and save what is left for your afternoon snack. Make sure to drink the whole batch from one recipe each day.

Morning snack: one small handful of any nuts, or roasted seed such as pumpkin seeds and sunflower seeds.

Lunch: salad with grilled chicken breast, salmon, or two boiled eggs. You may also add some beans, whole grains or sweet potatoes if needed. The recipes make a large batch, so eat just enough to feel satiated, and save any leftover for later.

Afternoon snack: Leftover smoothie

Dinner: vegetable stir-fry or soup.

Note: Remember to drink at least 8 glasses of water a day. Coffee is limited to 1 daily cup. Please do not go hungry. If in between the scheduled meals and snacks you still feel hungry, eat anything allowed on the plan, such as salad, smoothie, soup, a piece of fruits, nuts, or roasted seeds.

When making the recipes below, feel free to add any non-starchy vegetable that you like, or take out what you don't like. The food has to taste good for you, so make the needed adjustments.

Tips for Success:

- To start, select 10 smoothie recipes, making sure to include these two recipes: Tropical Turmeric Blast, and Blue-Pineapple.

- Look at the daily plan and recipes, and gather the ingredients for what you will be eating for at least five days. Doing so allows you to be prepared by having all what you need on hands, so you won't be tempted to eat foods that are not part of the plan.

- If you do not have time to make your smoothie in the morning, make it at night and refrigerate for the next day. You can also make smoothies for all 10 days and freeze, following the tips shared on pages 133 and 134.

- Grill the chicken breast and salmon, boil the eggs, prep the vegetables for the salad and save in the refrigerator. Also, make the salad dressing, or use any good brand of vinaigrette that you enjoy.

- Cook the soup and stir-fry, and refrigerate so you can have them ready when needed. It will last couple days, for the batches are large.

Romaine lettuce salad

- 2 cups chopped romaine lettuce
- 1/3 cup of sliced red onion
- ½ red bell pepper, seeded and sliced
- ½ cup cherry or grape tomatoes, halved
- 1 small cucumber or half a medium cucumber, cubed
- ¼ cup kalamata olives (optional)
- ½ avocado, cubed
- 1-2 garlic clove, crushed and minced
- ¼ cup parsley, chopped
- 1 piece of grilled chicken breast, or salmon, or 2 boiled eggs

Mix- greens salad

- 2 cups mix-greens
- 1/3 cup sliced red onion
- ½ red bell pepper, sliced
- ½ cup cherry or grape tomatoes, halved
- ¼ cup shredded carrot
- ¼ cup parsley or cilantro, chopped
- 1-2 garlic clove, crushed and minced
- ½ small avocado, cubed
- 1 grilled chicken breast, or salmon, or 2 boiled eggs

Power detox salad

- ½ cup red cabbage, shredded
- ½ cup green cabbage, shredded
- ½ cup carrot, shredded
- 1/3 cup sliced red onion
- 1/2 beet, shredded
- 1-2 garlic clove, crushed and minced
- ¼ cup cilantro, chopped
- ½ cup cherry or grape tomatoes, halved
- Salt and black pepper to taste
- 1 grilled chicken breast, or salmon, or 2 boiled eggs

Place cabbages in a bowl; add 1 tablespoon lemon juice or vinegar massage with your hands to soften. Place onion and garlic in a bowl, add some vinegar and let sit for about 5 minutes. Add all the other ingredients on the cabbage in layer; and then add salad dressing. Arrange chopped chicken breast or salmon on top and enjoy!

Dijon mustard vinaigrette

Ingredients:

- ½ cup extra virgin olive oil
- ¼ cup red wine vinegar
- 2 tsp Dijon mustard
- 1 tsp raw honey
- 1 garlic glove, crushed and minced
- ¼ tsp salt or to taste
- ¼ tsp black pepper or to taste

Directions:

This vinaigrette can be made in three different ways:

1. Beat the vinegar in a bowl with the honey, garlic, salt and pepper. Then add in the oil by droplets, whisking constantly.

2. You can place all the ingredients in a screw-top jar and shake to combine. Taste and adjust the seasonings.

3. Add all ingredients, but garlic and oil to a blender then blend until smooth. Add oil slowly when blender is still running. Continue to blend until smooth. Pour in a jar and add the garlic. Dressing can be store in the refrigerator for up to a week.

Grilled Chicken breast or salmon

Season some pieces of chicken breast or salmon with salt, black pepper and vinaigrette. Let rest in the refrigerator for at least two hours for chicken breast and only 30 minutes for salmon, and grill. Let cool and refrigerate in a bowl with lid. When ready for a salad, take out one piece, chop and add to your salad.

Super Detox Soup

Ingredients:

- ½ green cabbage, chopped
- ½ red cabbage, chopped
- 1 tablespoon extra-virgin olive oil
- 2 beets, diced
- 1 cup tomatoes, diced
- 2 carrots, diced

- 1 red onion, diced
- 1 can garbanzo beans, drained
- 8 ounces mushrooms, chopped
- 1 bell pepper, chopped (any color)
- 2 celery stalk, chopped
- 1 cup leek, chopped (including green and white part)
- 5 garlic gloves, crushed and minced
- 1 quart low sodium chicken or vegetable broth
- 1 bay leaf
- 1 tsp thyme
- Black pepper and salt to taste

Directions

Heat oil in a pan; add onions and sauté till the onions are translucent, and then add garlic and cook for one minute. Add the chopped veggies and beans. Stir well, and sauté on a medium flame for 4 to 5 minutes. Add the broth, thyme, bay leaf, black pepper and salt. Cover the pan and simmer the soup for 20-30 minutes or until ready, on a low to medium flame. Then check the seasonings and adjust as needed.

Stir-fry with herbs and mushrooms

Ingredients:

- 1 bag frozen carrot (about 12 ounces)
- 1 bag frozen green beans (about 12 ounces)
- 1 yellow squash
- 1 zucchini
- 1/2 green pepper
- 1/2 red pepper
- 8 ounces mushroom, sliced
- 1 cup onion, chopped
- 1 cup tomatoes, diced
- 3-4 garlic cloves, crushed, finely chopped
- 1/4 cup water or more as needed
- 1/4 cup basil, chopped (or 1 Tbsp. dry)
- ½ cup parsley, chopped) (or 2 Tbsp. dry)
- 1 Tbsp. fresh oregano, chopped (or 1 tsp. dry)
- 1-2 tsp. Bragg liquid aminos, or reduced sodium soy sauce, (I use Tamari soy sauce)
- Salt and black pepper to taste

Directions:

Heat the oil and add onions and cook for 3-4 minutes, then add garlic. Cook for 1-2 minutes, and then add the tomatoes. (If you are using dry herbs, add them now). Cook for about 3-5 minutes stirring often, and then add the carrot, green beans, mushrooms, the liquid aminos, or soy sauce, salt and pepper to taste. Continue stirring and add the water. Let cook until a little soft but not yet ready, stirring often, then add the zucchini, yellow squash, red and green peppers, and more salt and black pepper if needed. Continue stirring. If too dry add some water just a tablespoon at the time. If using fresh herb, when all the veggies are soft but just 1-2 minutes before completely ready, add the fresh herbs. Continue stirring until flavorful. Enjoy!

Note: You can also use Broccoli and Cauliflower, and leave out the green beans

Roasted seed

Ingredients:

- 1 cup sunflower seeds
- 1 cup pumpkin seeds
- 2-3 tsp. coconut or olive oil
- 1 tsp. paprika

- ½ tsp. cumin
- ½ tsp. salt
- ¼ tsp. black pepper
- ¼ tsp. cayenne pepper (optional)

Directions:

Preheat oven at 275 degree F (140 degree C). Mix all ingredients in a bowl, using your hands to make sure all the seeds are covered with oil and spices. Pour on a baking sheet in one layer, and bake for 5 minutes. Take out of oven and shake gently to move around. Return to the oven and continue baking for another 5 minutes. Take out, let cool and save in a glass jar with airtight lid.

Note: For a different flavor, you can also use 2 teaspoons of curry powder or any spice you like.

Wholesome Living Academy

Healthy Living God's way

www.wholesomelivingacademy.com

What we do:

We help women establish healthy eating and lifestyle habits and reach their health and wellness goals in the process.

Who we serve:

- Women who are looking for one-on-one, or group coaching support, to improve their health and maintain a healthy lifestyle.

- Women who want to lose weight and maintain it naturally, without relying on "yo-yo" dieting.

- Busy moms who are looking for convenient ways to create a healthy lifestyle for themselves and their families.

- Churches that are tired of seeing their members weakened by preventable chronic health conditions, such as obesity, heart disease, high blood pressure, Type 2 diabetes, and gastrointestinal disorders.

Services:

- Customized health and wellness coaching program for individuals and groups
- Healthy eating classes
- Healthy cooking classes
- Healthy living classes
- Workshops
- Speaking engagement on health and wellness

Contact us to learn more:
www.wholesomelivingacademy.com

Uplift Your Health and Beauty With Our High Protein Collagen Shake

How can Collagen help you?

Among other health benefits, collagen may help:

- Minimize fine lines and wrinkles
- Promote skin elasticity and firmness
- Support strong hair, and nails
- Support join comfort and mobility, by reducing inflammation and pain
- Reduce discomfort associated with IBS, and other gastrointestinal disorders, and support the healing of leaking gut
- Support wound healing

Radiant Beauty, from inside out!

Check out www.upliftingfoods.com to learn more

For ongoing motivation, health tips and recipes,

Follow Nathalie Talom on social media:

Facebook

YouTube

Twitter

Instagram

Visit her websites where you can subscribe to her blog:

www.upliftingfoods.com

www.wholesomelivingacademy.com

Let's get back to nature and reclaim our health!

NOTES

Author's Note

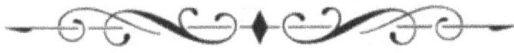

I am originally from Cameroon where I grew up before immigrating to the United States. Early in my life I came to experience the healing power of nature, as in Cameroon it is common to consume a variety of plants, including herbs, roots, and spices for their health benefits. This practice is even more intensified in rural areas where medical care is limited.

The first time I visited my grandfather in the village, I was amazed by his knowledge of herbal medicine. One of his hobbies was to create different concoctions to help people manage certain ailments. He had a garden in his backyard where he grew a variety of medicinal plants, and in his kitchen, there was a special grinding stone that was only used for those plants. Consuming some of these medicinal plants daily was part of his normal routine, whether he was sick or not. He was convinced that they had defensive compounds that protected people from certain diseases, as well as boosted vitality.

I rarely heard that my grandfather was sick. While he may have caught a bug now and then, it was never serious enough to put him in the hospital. He was 99 years old when he died, and was still walking miles a day without a cane, had a good memory, and was on no medications. His father, who had the same lifestyle, died at 100+ years.

All things considered, as I thought about my grandfather's life, I realized that his consistent intake of plant foods, along with other health promoting habits, such as adequate rest and activity, went a long way toward contributing to his good health and longevity. Looking at other traditional cultures around the world, I noticed a similar lifestyle pattern in people experiencing good health. In our modern-day society, however, we tend to rely mainly on pills. Sadly those pills are not always the best answer, and often come with side effects that might require new pills; leading people to a trap of medications dependency.

Consuming a variety of plants foods with known health benefits either for prevention or as part of a treatment regimen, is not something most people think about. This observation has promoted my passion for helping people to reconnect with nature, through the consumption of high quality, nourishing and healing foods. My mission is to look around the world, for those foods that people have successfully used to nourish their bodies and promote health. It is my desire to introduce those superfoods in our western diet, in as easy and convenient a way as possible, so anyone can enjoy the benefits of good health, vitality, and longevity. For this reason, I founded Uplifting Foods, a health food company dedicated to fostering a healthy life experience. Check us out at:

www.upliftingfoods.com

www.ingramcontent.com/pod-product-compliance
Lightning Source LLC
Chambersburg PA
CBHW061015280326
41935CB00009B/972